T0375206

RECLAIM YOUR STRENGTH AND HOPE

EXERCISES FOR CANCER CORE RECOVERY®

Foreword by Kris Carr, New York Times best-selling
author, Wellness Advocate and Cancer Thriver

ILANA CASS, MD, CHAIR OF OBSTETRICS & GYNECOLOGY AT GEISEL SCHOOL
OF MEDICINE, DARTMOUTH-HITCHCOCK
PROFESSOR OBSTETRICS AND GYNECOLOGY, CEDARS SINAI MEDICAL
CENTER

"Emilee shows women how to rebuild, refocus, and emerge stronger in a truly gentle and caring way. Her exercises are safe, gradual steps that women can do from their hospital beds to their own bedrooms to build endurance, confidence, and strength. It's "progress, not perfection," and Emilee's book is there at your side along the journey to feeling whole again."

Emilee Garfield

BALBOA.
PRESS
A DIVISION OF HAY HOUSE

Balboa Press books may be ordered through booksellers or by contacting:

Balboa Press
A Division of Hay House
1663 Liberty Drive
Bloomington, IN 47403
www.balboapress.com
1 (877) 407-4847

Print information available on the last page.

ISBN: 978-1-9822-2615-2 (sc)
ISBN: 978-1-9822-2614-5 (hc)
ISBN: 978-1-9822-2620-6 (e)

Library of Congress Control Number: 2019904466

Balboa Press rev. date: 08/23/2019

Disclaimer

Consult a physician before performing this or any exercise program. It is your responsibility to evaluate your own medical and physical condition, or that of your clients, and to independently determine whether to perform, use, or adapt any of the information or content in this book or in videos on YouTube.

Any exercise program may result in injury. By voluntarily undertaking any exercise displayed, you assume the risk of any resulting injury.

Emilee Garfield specifically disclaims liability for incidental or consequential damages and assumes no responsibility or liability for any loss or damage suffered by any person as a result of the use or misuse of any of the information or content in the *Reclaim Your Strength and Hope: Exercises for Cancer Core Recovery* book.

Visit Emilee's website for further information and exercise resources to improve your quality of life during recovery: www.emileegarfield.com

Contents

Foreword BY KRIS CARR
Author of *Crazy Sexy Cancer*

Over a decade ago, I was diagnosed with an incurable, stage IV cancer.

Since you're reading Emilee's stellar guide to recovering and restoring your beautiful body (smart cookie!), you know what a total shocker it is to hear that kind of news.

At the time, it felt like a tidal wave of fear swept through my life and I was being pulled under. But really, it was my wake-up call to live a life filled to the brim with intention and purpose. I realized that the only person who could help me was me. So I became the CEO of my life and took control of my own wellness.

I began living mindfully and healthfully. This included adopting a plant-based diet, drinking delicious green drinks, and smoothing and zen-ing out with meditation each morning.

Exercise was also added to my non-negotiable list. Let's just say movement plays a major part in protecting your ass-ets!

Besides the obvious health benefits, exercise also increases your level of endorphins, dopamine, and serotonin, which helps you feel more joyful, relaxed, and clear-minded.

After meeting Emilee during a session of B-School, I ordered her workout DVD and asked to have a peek at her upcoming exercise guide. I absolutely loved it, and you will too!

In *Reclaim Your Strength and Hope: Exercises for Cancer Core Recovery,* Emilee gives you the keys to gently and safely stretch all major muscle groups and strengthen your core.

She compassionately walks you through each phase of recovery—it's like she's right by your side, coaching you along the way. Plus, her personality is upbeat, fun, and inspirational—which will help you stay oh-so-motivated. From one cancer patient to another, I can honestly say that Emilee is a treasure.

To have someone who has undergone the same experiences with cancer—even though it's unique for everyone—is a gift. I felt she connected with me and understood the vulnerabilities of being a cancer survivor.

Not only does this guide include exercises, but it also has gorgeous coloring pages, soulful journal prompts, and inspiring advice for those days when the most you can do is roll over in your bed and pick up a book!

From phase 1 exercises that you can do in your hospital bed, all the way to phase 5 advanced strengthening and balance exercises, Emilee will inspire you to move, even if it's only sitting up in a chair for a few seconds or walking across a room.

She organized this guide to be followed from the start of your recovery in your hospital bed to the moment you are standing on your feet at home. You can't go wrong with her method of taking you through each phase, s-l-o-w-l-y. The beautiful thing is that you won't overdo it during recovery.

A slow and steady recovery means lifelong healing and good health.

Do not rush through your exercises, or any aspect of your healing journey, for that matter. We live in a culture that's obsessed with quick fixes. I encourage you to savor every moment of your life and to see how beautiful you are, right now.

Emilee believes that cancer recovery is a process, not a race to the finish line toward a beach-perfect body. I love her philosophy and this guide too!

You will treasure it for years to come, perhaps even years after recovery. The exercise gems in *Reclaim Your Strength and Hope* can be enjoyed by all fitness levels.

Remember to keep moving and grooving that gorgeous body of yours. You are so worth it!

Peace and slow-like-honey healing,
Kris Carr
New York Times **best-selling author**

Advance Praise

As a gynecological surgeon, I know that this isn't easy territory. Surgery, recovery in a hospital, and then the cancer treatments can all conspire to rob women of any sense of control over their bodies.

Emilee shows women how to rebuild, refocus, and emerge stronger in a truly gentle and caring way. Her exercises are safe, gradual steps that women can do from their hospital beds to their own bedrooms to build endurance, confidence, and strength. It's "progress, not perfection," and Emilee's book is there at your side along the journey to feeling whole again.

I wholeheartedly endorse Emilee's cancer recovery plan and her spirit embodied in this unique book for women.

—Ilana Cass, professor of obstetrics and gynecology, Gynecologic Oncology, Cedars Sinai Medical Center

Emilee has written a book that is perfect for all patients undergoing abdominal or pelvic surgery. Through her own experience, she has realized that recovery from surgery is not a race, but a journey. She embodies mind, body, and spirit to a successful restoration of excellent health. Emilee elicits safe and dependable mental and physical exercises for a solid core recovery. I will recommend this book to all my patients.

—Beth Moore, MD, colorectal surgeon, Cedars Sinai Medical Center

Emilee's book is unique in that it's designed for cancer survivors who have had lower abdominal surgeries, yet anyone who needs to strengthen his or her core can get so much out of it.

Her understanding of the dynamic movement of the body and how to strengthen from the core is amazing.

Her guide is effective for safely and gently stretching and strengthening the whole body. I recommend it to all of my patients.

—Jason Snibbe, MD, Orthopedic Hip Institute. Beverly Hills

One afternoon in 2016, Emilee sat down on my patio to talk about her Cancer Core Recovery® Project. She had a sparkle in her eyes and a big smiley face. Boundless energy and motivation radiated all around her.

I knew then and there that she embodied survival in the most powerful and vibrant way.

Immediately, she told me her story, introduced her project ideas, and added, "Look, I have no time to waste! I need to get this out there."

She didn't waste a moment. Still, she wrote this book in the most thoughtful and thorough manner, with a tenacity not unlike her own recovery.

Emilee's book projects her brilliance: it is filled with wit and written with honesty, compassion, and encouragement to coach the reader through every phase of his or her recovery.

Her expertise as a movement educator in yoga and Pilates for over 21 years is well represented in this book. Combined with her real life experience of cancer recovery that she openly shares, this book shines with Emilee's self-confidence, renewed energy, and unshakeable hope, which has been captured on every page.

Each recovery phase is carefully planned and richly illustrated. Every stretch and exercise sequence is clearly explained. The notes of encouragement do not leave even the smallest pitfalls out.

What makes *Reclaim Your Strength and Hope* so unique is the fact that there is no other book on the market that safely coaches your recovery from day one—while still in the hospital bed!

The survivor will not be the only one to benefit from this book. Thanks to Emilee sharing her true feelings and mindset of the survivor during the recovery process, this book will become an essential read and guide for the doctor, caregiver, and movement educator alike.

Thank you, Emilee, for your book and for your inspiration.

—Marie-José Blom, creator and president of SmartSpine Wellness System

Recently, I had the pleasure of participating in Emilee Garfield's Cancer Core Recovery® class.

Members of my urology team, my husband, and my four-week-old newborn joined Emilee for a session. Our group of participants could not have been more diverse in regards to fitness levels and prior life events.

Emilee challenged all of us in a safe and effective manner in addition to inspiring and motivating us, both as individuals and a team.

We had a blast optimizing ourselves with Emilee, who successfully battled a rhabdomyosarcoma pelvic tumor as a child and stage 111C ovarian cancer as an adult!

I commend Emilee for developing a mental and physical recovery program for patients after significant abdominal or pelvic surgery. As a urologist who focuses on pelvic wellness, I can affirm the need for such a positive recovery program after urologic treatments for cancer and other pathologies. Emilee's book *Reclaim Your Strength and Hope: Exercises for Cancer Core Recovery* fills this void.

Patients will greatly benefit spiritually and physically from Emilee's Cancer Core Recovery® program! Her never-quit attitude and "go big or go home" philosophy will facilitate others to be the best version of themselves during challenging times.

—Alex Rogers, MD Urology, Santa Barbara

To all of you who have had cancer and/or are recovering from major abdominal surgery, I dedicate this book to you.

I dedicate this book to my kids Hayden, Griffin, and Macie, who reminded me that I can't quit, because I told them to never give up. My kids are my everything.

Thank you, thank you, thank you, to my mom, who dropped her life to come live with me for eight months and help take care of me and my kids.

Thank you ...

To all of you who joined me on this crazy journey, for never giving up on me.

To my best friend, Mark, for telling me I was beautiful every day, even when I didn't feel beautiful and for being my angel that never left my side. You were there for me 100% of the way! And, thank you for rubbing my feet in the hospital and helping me believe I was stronger than I thought.

Kris, my amazing copywriter and friend, for sticking by my side through blood, sweat, and tears to get this project completed. During this process, we went through many heartbreaks together: divorces and the loss of your mom from pancreatic cancer. I know she is looking down from heaven and cheering that we finally got this finished.

All of my doctors for working as a team to save my life so that I could spread hope and joy to others following in my shoes.

Dr. Fred Kass for saving lives, especially mine and showing me how to have humor through it all.

A special thanks to **Dr. Ilana Cass** for telling me that my cancer was GO BIG or GO HOME and that I had three beautiful kids to fight for.

Terri Weissglass for creating the gorgeous journaling pictures and prompts.

Fit Life Productions for donating your time and efforts to create all the workout and educational videos for the Cancer Core Recovery® Project.

EMILEE GARFIELD

Marie-José Blom for sitting with me on your patio and listening when I first showed you my project. I was so afraid, but you smiled and told me that I had a great project to share.

Laura Horn for guiding me with your professional knowledge of pelvic wellness and women's health.

Dr. Alex Rodgers, my favorite urologist, for testing and trying out these exercises with your medical staff. Thank you for trusting me and acknowledging the need for this book.

Alecia & Aija Mayrock for believing in me and pushing me to write this book. Best Selling author of *The Survival Guide to Bullying*.

Nancy Levin for helping me love myself and see my worth. Best Selling Author of *Worthy* and *Jump and Your Life Will Appear*.

This book was created for you so that you do not walk this path alone. I am right here with you all of the way. Thank you.

Introduction

Hello, beautiful.

These two words stuck by me throughout my cancer journey, and it was because of a friend texting me every day saying, "Good morning, beautiful" and "Hello, beautiful."

His words helped me to get out of bed every day and move my body. I want to pass on these healing words to encourage you during your recovery.

I didn't feel beautiful, so these messages meant the world to me. I wanted to live. I wanted a fresh start.

And I wanted to feel beautiful in my own skin.

Welcome to the journey. Know that you are not alone. We are in this together.

I'm so excited you picked up this survival guide—nope, actually, it's a *thrival* guide. It is so much more than just a book of exercises.

In the beginning, I designed this book for women like me with ovarian cancer, but then I noticed that there were many others that could benefit as well.

Your caretaker can even do this recovery program with you!

Fun, right?

Everything in here is easy to do. For those times when nothing feels easy (which happened a lot for me), I offer you modifications that will match your energy level.

Although these exercises are inspired by yoga and Pilates, you don't need to have prior experience with either. I'll teach you my methods from start to finish.

I know you want your energetic, active life back and your body back, but please, please hear me out. Healing is a process, and if you rush it, you will have a setback. Believe me, that's the last thing you want.

As you follow this guidebook of core exercises and stretches, you will notice it's organized into phases. You might look at them and say, "That looks too easy!" Or, "I used to do yoga or Zumba or Pilates class, and I want to go back to my old routine." I said the same thing.

I'm not trying to sound negative, but here's the truth that I've experienced firsthand: your body is not the same. Listen to your body when it says, "Slow down."

If you start to move and think of your body in a new way, you will surprise yourself at how easily you can learn to love and appreciate your body even more than before you had cancer.

I will be with you 100 percent of the way.

And don't let the word *core* fool you. Just so you know, this is not a "work your six-pack abs" sort of exercise program—and you're not doing plank push-ups either.

In this book, I will teach you exercises for core recovery, so you can discover and use your deep core muscles that will make you strong from the inside out. These muscles are vital to learning how to rehabilitate after surgery. They will help you with side effects from surgery and radiation (including incontinence, lower limb lymphedema and just straight-out back pain).

Trust me, I would never teach you something that I hadn't done myself. The last thing I want is for you to be in more pain.

Of course, you may have fear of injuring your body by stretching and moving! I completely understand. I have been there too.

Luckily for me, my profession was and still is educating and teaching Pilates and yoga. I'm a movement educator that teaches movement as medicine! I had cancer as a child, so my body had already been through this once.

It's the old saying, "This isn't my first rodeo"—and, well, that's the truth. This time around, I was old enough and educated to know that I could change my mindset and take control of my body.

In my own recovery process, I simply started by waking up each morning, crawling out of bed, progressing toward stretching my body using my own bed and kitchen sink, and eventually walking around the house.

Sounds easy, right?

It wasn't.

There were days when rolling to my side in bed was the most I could motivate myself to do.

Yep, start with the simplest routines and eventually work your way up to the later exercises in this manual.

How to Use This Book

The exercises in phase 1 include very gentle stretches and movements that stimulate blood flow. Your recovery begins in the hospital, and the sooner you start moving, the sooner you will get out of the hospital and back to your life. Don't get mad at your nurse when she tells you to get up and walk! It's the best thing you can do for yourself.

Please don't be in a hurry to jump back into your old routine. I put my heart and soul into writing *every* single exercise I did at *each* phase of my recovery. I'm so excited to share these with you!

In the beginning, if you had abdominal surgery like I did, your abdomen is still swollen and you have stitches and maybe a new ostomy like me. You may be in *shock* at what your new body looks like, but you *will* get through it.

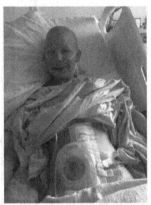

Follow the book from the beginning to the end. I'll take you on a journey. At first, it's all about relaxing.

The good news is that there is no rush, there is no timeline, and we all heal differently. There is no one right way, so I want you to know that you can't fail at this. I made it failure-proof.

If you feel scared or nervous, ask your nurse or caretaker to do the exercises with you. You'll be surprised to find that he or she enjoys doing the stretches as much as you do.

Phase 1 of this book is done while you're recovering in the hospital. These include simple exercises in bed where you bend your knees and stretch your feet. At the end of this phase, you'll be on your way to sitting in a chair. Don't beat yourself up if you don't have the energy to do all of phase 1 in the hospital. You can start after you return home and feel ready.

You can pick and choose the exercises that feel right for you.

By the way, if you had breast surgery, you will need to modify the exercises and be gentle with your arms. I didn't have surgery on or near my arms, so I didn't have to be as careful as you. If the arm exercises really feel uncomfortable, skip them altogether.

In phase 2, you will begin your exercises at home. I've tried to make it as simple as possible for you. What you'll be doing is not traditional yoga or Pilates; it's my own recipe for rehabilitating your body in the safest way possible.

When you are feeling lazy and have been on the couch for too long, try to remember this: sitting is the new smoking. Get up and walk around the house. Sitting on your butt for too long is not going to help you recover quickly. Walking will.

Walking is by far the best way to begin your recovery program. On a side note, it also increases lymph flow so all the toxins drain out. Think of the lymphatic system as your body's own garbage disposal!

Movement will help prevent something your doctor may not have told you about–lower limb lymphedema. Basically, this means swelling of the legs. It's now known that it can occur many years after your original surgery—up to ten years later! This is why I slowly marched my legs in bed. (Check this out in phase 2. The exercise is called Simple Knee Lift.)

Before you begin phase 3, make sure your tummy is all healed up and you are about six to eight weeks post-surgery, maybe even longer if you're getting used to your new ostomy. Listen to your body, and don't beat yourself up if you need extra time to get ready for this phase. Of course, you should always get your doctor's clearance first.

Begin when you no longer have intense pain in your abdomen. It's normal to feel tight inside from the scar tissue, but hopefully the prior phases have helped you stretch out and you're able to hold yourself up tall again.

Phase 3 is the central part of my exercise program that uses my unique methods of rebuilding strength in your deep core muscles. You can safely begin this section of the guide when you feel healed in your abdomen and are ready to move to the next step.

I love this phase and you will too! It takes the fear out of exercising your core. One of the benefits of strengthening your core is decreased back pain. I created it for myself because there was nothing out there to address the kind of recovery I was going through!

At first, I didn't care how my body looked; I just wanted to function without being in pain. Scar tissue inside the surgical site was *so* painful.

I realized that healing my body was going to be a process.

After radiation damaged and weakened the tissues in my abdomen and pelvis, I lost sensation inside my core. I had to slow down, listen to my body, and let it teach me.

I modified a lot because of my ileostomy. I created this routine for myself because of my limited range of movement. If I tried to do a regular workout, it just didn't happen, and I got frustrated. I also developed body-image issues, and the last thing I wanted to do was judge myself.

In phase 3, you will need to use 2 small, 10" stability balls. They allow you to feel safe and supported. You will be able to find a deeper part of your core muscles by using the balls. You will be amazed at how much you will feel with these little movements.

It felt amazing when I did a series of poses called "chest openers." I could feel the scar tissue gently stretching in my belly. I can't wait to share these exercises with you!

Be mindful and concentrate on timing and micro-mini movements to strengthen your body on a deeper level.

This is what makes these exercises so unique and perfect for anyone who needs to rebuild their core muscles.

Slow down and work deeper, not bigger.

In phase 4, we'll focus on regaining your balance. Having a strong core will help you develop better balance.

Once you get to the final section, phase 5, you're ready for more advanced strengthening movements.

The timeline for each of the phases completely depends on your body's recovery needs.

My hope is that you walk away with at least this *one* thing from reading this book; it's learning to **slow down and listen to your body**.

Listen to your breath. Your body is always trying to teach you something … listen.

Movement is medicine.

Video Downloads

Nearly all of the exercises in this book have matching instructional videos on YouTube.

Visit my YouTube channel to get the exercises from this book. These are the essentials to get you started:

http://bit.ly/CancerCoreExercises

You can continue the journey with me and get the full benefits of learning many more exercises that I did in my own recovery by taking my online course, **Exercises for Cancer Core Recovery.**

The course includes 100+ easy to follow instructional videos that will help you rebuild strength, balance and flexibility. I'll be with you the whole way, cheering you on and inspiring you to reclaim your hope and joy!

To find all of my programs and courses, visit my website at www. emileegarfield.com.

I'm A Survivor

I am strong.
I am resilient. I try my best.
I value my life.
I am not perfect, but I am the perfect me.
I never give up.
I am empathetic.
I am a warrior, ready to conquer.
I am not broken.
I am loving.
I take things one day at a time.
I am independent.
I am human.
I am a survivor.
                    —Author unknown

My Journey with Cancer

I always tell people, "Cancer saved my life."

For many people cancer can take them down, and the thing was that I was already as far down as I could go. I had lost hope for living and lost myself in the process. I had hit rock bottom and the only way to go was up. Then, the cancer diagnosis.

We all deal with our cancer diagnosis differently. For me, cancer was my BIG wake up call.

Cancer saved my life.

This project saved my life. It kept me focused on having a purpose in life, which is to help others with cancer.

Before the diagnosis, I felt unlovable, worthless and alone. I was afraid nobody would ever love me because of the way I looked after all of my surgeries, but that wasn't true.

Cancer has taught me that I am worth living for and that there are others out there who need my help because they might feel like I did. I'm here to tell you that even if you feel hopeless and aren't sure if you have the strength to fight cancer, YOU DO.

I remember an appointment with my surgeon when she told me that my Stage 3C ovarian cancer was "nasty" and I was going to lose part of my colon and my "girly parts," which she could partially reconstruct from my abs. I burst into tears.

I couldn't believe that I had to fight cancer a second time. When she showed me what my new body would look like, I told her, "I'd rather die." She reminded me that I had three gorgeous kids to live for. That was the first time I had hope that I could survive cancer.

Post-operation: I woke up with a colon bag and catheter that I later dragged around in a pillowcase. I didn't want to leave the house. I felt ashamed. I know how hard it is to talk about cancer of the "girly parts." Now I'm on a mission to help other women thrive during cancer recovery, particularly those who have suffered from gynecological cancers.

I decided to fight. I chose to live. I chose me.

Cancer would not control my destiny. I realized how I needed to change my story—and took my power back. Believe me, if I could do it, so can you. We all have a comeback story to tell because we've all lost ourselves at some point in our lives.

While struggling with a new ileostomy, incontinence, and internal tissue damage from previous cancer surgeries and radiation (from as far back as my early childhood), I returned to work as a Pilates, yoga and movement educator.

I was frustrated to find limited resources locally about how to exercise safely with an ostomy. After teaching Pilates and yoga and working as a movement educator for eighteen years, I understand the human body. I was aware that movement was essential for my recovery and improving my quality of life. I knew movement would be my medicine.

I created my own recovery program to get back on my feet. These methods became my signature Cancer Core Recovery® exercise programs that I teach to other cancer survivors and the medical professionals who treat them.

In 2017, I created my foundation, the **Cancer Core Recovery® Project,** a 501 (c)(3) non-profit organization with this mission: to help women recovering from ovarian cancer overcome their bodies' new limitations post-surgery and treatment so they can live a better quality of life.

My mission is helping women reclaim their strength and hope using movement as medicine.

I show people how to see the good in themselves and how miraculous they are. I always tell them, "Never give up!" Live life full of joy and hope.

Whether your scars are visible or invisible, both are equally debilitating. No matter where you are now or how awful things are, there is always a way to the next level of feeling better. Sometimes you get there inch by inch, but you will get there!

Change is a process, not a race to the finish line. You can trust that I will be there each step of the way, cheering you on!

My passion in life has been teaching people how to love and honor their bodies, no matter what. In order to create change in our lives and the healthy bodies we need, we must show up and do the work. Real, lasting change must be embodied through taking action.

My dream is to continue to inspire, encourage, and motivate you through my words, my coaching, and my teaching for many years to come.

The most empowering advice that I can give you right now: Love and respect your body. Be kind to yourself. You are worth it.

I hope the story of my cancer journey inspires you and gives you hope for what's possible.

My Motivational Speech
(For When You're Ready to Give Up)

Read this out loud on those days when you feel like quitting or when you don't have the motivation to get up and move.

I got this.

That voice is a liar.

I can do this, and I will do this.

I can get up and move my body, even for just five minutes. Because movement is medicine.

It may be hard, but I am not afraid of hard. Because I am worthy. I got this!

I deserve joy, radiant health and respect.

Love and Hugs

Thank you.

If it weren't for you, this book would not have been written.

These exercises would have stayed locked up inside me and would not be passed on and shared for your healing and the benefit of others.

Follow my guide, and please *relax* in the beginning. I am so thankful that I practiced yoga and knew the benefits of certain yoga poses. I modified them to create stretches that felt good for my pelvis and abdomen.

We are all unique. My story is different from yours, but I know these exercises will help you get back into your life so that you too can be jumping for joy!

Now, it's your turn! Get up and go … unless you're in bed, in which case, start doing those heel slides!

Gratitude is the holy grail of healing.

So, again, with deep bows of gratitude and respect—thank you from the bottom of my heart!

With all my love,
Emilee ♥

Self-Care: Coloring Pages and Journal Prompts to Inspire Joy

I want to share a few of my favorite things that I used that helped lift my spirits when I was in a funk.

Playing in my coloring books and journaling while waiting for office visits and chemotherapy treatments helped ease my anxieties and fears.

My hope is that this self-care section will bring you some comfort as well.

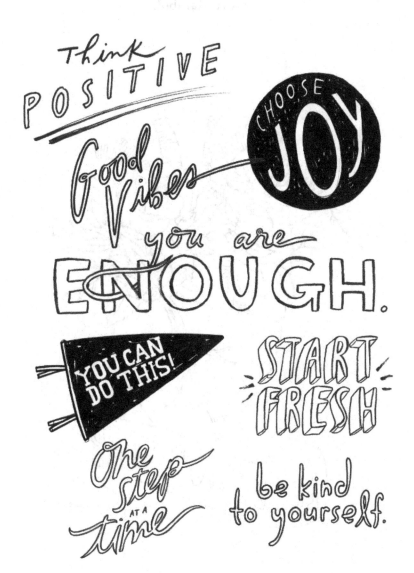

We all have scars, both visible and invisible. Remind yourself today that scars are beautiful and they tell your unique story.

"My scars tell a story. They are a reminder of times when life tried to break me, but failed. They are markings of where the structure of my character was welded."
- **Steve Maraboli**

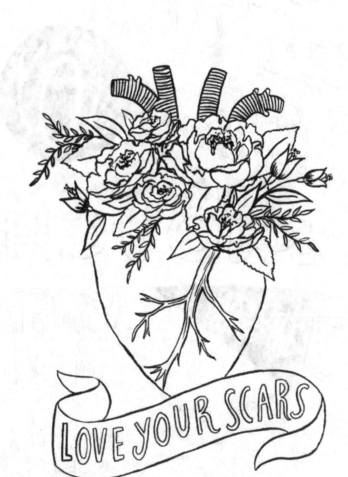

Close your eyes and picture yourself standing in a sunny field of flowers. Pick your favorites, breathe in, and imagine how fragrant they smell.

Enjoy coloring these flowers for your personal bouquet!

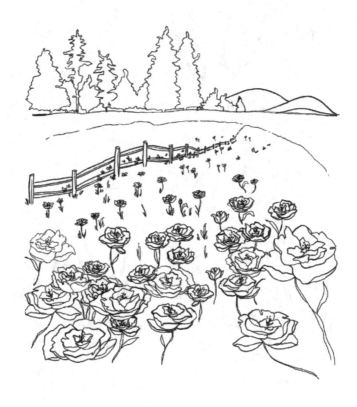

Close your eyes and imagine walking along the ocean shore. What do you see, hear?

Enjoy coloring these shells and sea life as wildly as you wish!

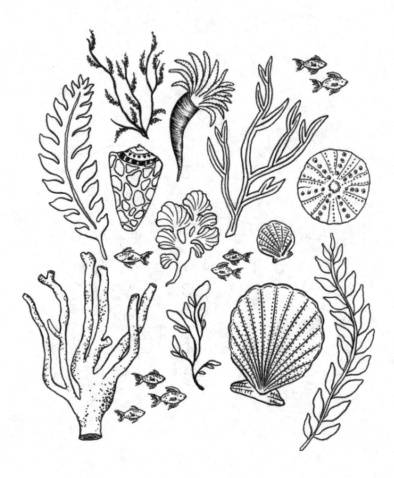

Close your eyes and imagine sitting atop a mountain on a warm evening, watching a beautiful sunset.

Enjoy creating your very own, amazing sunset with vibrant colors!

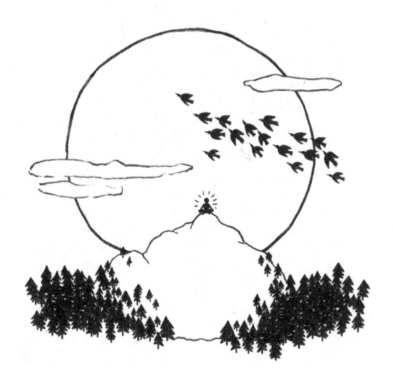

Close your eyes and picture yourself laughing with a few of your favorite people and/or animal companions!

Write your name in the center heart. Then beam out your incandescent joy as you write their names in the other hearts.

Color each heart brightly for a picture of the deep love that you richly deserve!

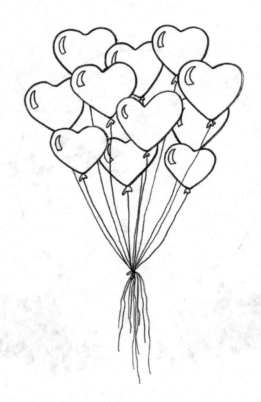

Positive Mindset Practices to Heal From The Inside Out

When you are recovering from cancer you have one job only.

Your job now is to do whatever it takes to create a more happy and joyful state of being. Period.

I know that this is going to be a challenge because I went through the same process!

Don't forget that **healing is a process**. It's not linear. Every day of my recovery I reminded myself that I was ALIVE! That led me to feel grateful for everything, including my lower back pain, which was excruciating nearly every day.

The bad news is that one day you may feel 100% better and the next you may wonder how you could feel so awful *again*.

The good news is that your recovery experience is unique to you and you are infinitely powerful. You can improve your well-being through the power of your mind and spirit. You can't control the outside world and outer circumstances of your life. You absolutely can control your mind and your reactions to those circumstances.

I wrote this book so you could heal both your mind and your body––you can't have one without the other. When your mind and body are connected, powerful healing occurs. I saw this for myself in my own recovery.

I believe it helps your healing process to focus on living, not on dying, one of our biggest fears. Negative thoughts can consume you and make you feel even more depressed and hopeless. Try shifting your mindset to living every day like it matters. You can find joy even in the hardest times of your life, like going through cancer.

Here are three questions that really helped me shift my mindset during my recovery. Pull out your journal or a notebook and write down the answers to these questions for yourself:

What would it be like if you looked at your recovery as a game?

What if you could be playful and curious about your body while healing from cancer?

What if you took this opportunity to learn something new about yourself and your body?

Try revisiting these journal questions again in three months and see how your thoughts have shifted and life has transformed.

Recovering from cancer can teach us a lot about ourselves, emotionally and physically. You never know how strong you are until you have to be.

Everyone deals with cancer differently. It was my second go at it and I told myself that this time I wasn't going to let cancer take my power away, like it did when I was a child. This time I wanted to be in control. I knew I had to become my own hero. You can become the hero of your own life and take your story back into your hands.

During my recovery, I played a mind game that helped me to shift the negative thoughts and feelings to more positive ones. Whenever a negative thought would flash through my mind, such as "I'm going to die," I would take a deep breath in and create a statement that was the opposite: "I will survive." I wouldn't let myself get too far into the future.

I would focus on the present. I reminded myself that, "Today is all I have." That is something that helped me go the distance. I didn't concentrate on the "what if," I focused on living for today and now. It helped me stay positive in a dark and uncertain situation.

What negative statement keeps coming up for you?

Now, try to create a more positive statement out of that negative thought. Use it as a mantra that you can repeat all day.

I tried to find the positive in the negative every day. That doesn't mean that I was 100% percent happy every day. I am human. I had some really hard days. Honestly, I had more hard days than good ones. Most days I felt like I was drowning from the overwhelm of anxiety, fear and sadness I felt. But, I got through them and you will too.

I chose to embrace as much as possible. I took life day by day and enjoyed the simple things like going for a walk and breathing fresh air.

Writing in my journal every day for 5 minutes brought much needed perspective to my life. I was going through a divorce, losing my house, financially broke and uncertain how I would take care of my three young kids. It was the perfect storm. But through it all, I maintained a force of strength that I never knew I had. I have no idea where it came from, but when I needed it, it came.

Trust the universe. Trust your faith. Trust that things will work out for the best.

Trust in you.

The journey can be as sad or as uplifting as you want to make it. Try to see the silver lining throughout your cancer journey.

One of my big silver linings was meeting positive, uplifting friends who truly cared about me and who helped me to laugh at life more often.

People look at me weird when I tell them that *cancer saved my life*, but my healing and wounds go much deeper than the physical body. I am sure you have some healing inside there to do, too. I think we all do. Take this time for yourself. Love yourself, respect yourself and heal those old wounds. I looked at cancer as a little vacation to heal the old and bring in the new. This is how I began to create my new life. The new and improved me. I met a 94-year old man named Ken who has taught me that I matter and that loving yourself is the first step in healing.

The next story I am going to share with you happened at the time I thought my life was a disaster. I couldn't see the light at the end of the tunnel. Everyday something bad would happen to me. It felt like I was cursed. But after a while, I started to laugh at myself because it just didn't seem possible that one person could take on so much pain and so many challenges.

Look, I am here now writing to you! I got through it. I can look back now and laugh at some of these stories. Laughter was the best medicine for me and still is. I hope you have a lot of good laughs too. Remember, you are stronger than you think you are.

Blowout on 405 Freeway

One day on the 405 freeway in Los Angeles, I had a blow out and it wasn't my tire.

I was on my way to Cedars Sinai hospital with my mom to go to my radiology appointment.

As I was sitting in traffic with my mom, I suddenly felt a burst of cold fluids coming down my stomach and leg. I looked down and said, *"WTF!"* I was just getting used to my new ileostomy and went into panic. I cried. I got mad. My mom and I got into a fight. But eventually, I laughed at the things I couldn't control.

There was nowhere to pull over so I sat in bumper to bumper traffic with liquid "poop" in my pants until we arrived at the hospital. My mom and I had to laugh! There was absolutely nothing we could do.

When we arrived, I got out of my car holding my stomach and panty area praying to God that nothing would leave a trail behind me. As soon as I made it to the bathroom, I pulled off my pants which were destroyed.

Since I forgot my change of clothes, I had to clean off my pants and put them back on damp and all. I was mortified.

After I cleaned myself up, I hobbled over to the nurse's station with paper towels around my stoma (where you attach the ileostomy bag). It felt like I was holding onto an alien. I had no control over my body.

I hope you're having a good laugh from reading that story! Yes, the situation was painful, frustrating and embarrassing. But that's life, so why not take things a bit more lightly?

Laughter is the best medicine, right?! It is one of the easiest ways to shift your mindset when things feel really … crappy!

What brings you the most joy in your life right now? Who or what makes you laugh the most?

Make it a point to surround yourself with people, places and things that uplift your spirit and put a smile on your face.

Honestly, keeping a positive mindset was one of the most challenging things I had to do during my recovery. It seemed silly. "I have CANCER. How can I tell my mind to be happy? How can I change my thoughts?" Trust me, if I can do it, anyone can.

People told me to meditate, which was hard because I'm not good at sitting still. My anxiety and my mind were completely wild and out of control! There were so many thoughts going through my head. Literally, I did anything to get my mind to settle so I wouldn't feel panicked and afraid.

The easiest way to get my thoughts out of my head was to journal. I began blogging on my Caring Bridge website. Even if no one was reading them, it helped me to express myself.

I practiced yoga and Pilates movements that I modified for myself, since I had an ileostomy (that's how the Cancer Core Recovery® Method was born). I walked around the block. Some days I could only walk for five minutes at the most. Doing the littlest things, even just walking a few steps a day if that's all you have in you, will accumulate and help you heal and rebuild your strength faster.

In the next few pages, I will share the practices I did during my own recovery, which I still do to this day!

Gratitude is Powerful Medicine

"I truly believe we can either see the connections, celebrate them, and express gratitude for our blessings, or we can see life as a string of coincidences that have no meaning or connection. For me, I'm going to believe in miracles, celebrate life, rejoice in the views of eternity, and hope my choices will create a positive ripple effect in the lives of others. This is my choice." **- Mike Ericksen**

One of the most healing practices you can try during your recovery process is to remember what you have to be GRATEFUL for. It sounds so simple and it's still the most powerful way to increase your joy and happiness.

Once you get in the habit of remembering what you're grateful for each day, you will find that your healing process feels more joyful and fun!

Here's a flashback for you. I wrote this piece about "gratitude" on July 15, 2015 while I was still in the hospital:

10 Things I Am Grateful For Today

1. **Having gas-ha!** Making fart sounds. The nurse said it's awesome I'm making gas or farting sounds. You may not know it, but passing gas and making fart sounds is the first thing the doctors listen for at the hospital. It means things are working inside your body.

2. **My lungs/oxygen**. It's something we take for granted. After wearing an oxygen mask on my face for the first 3 days I never realized how good fresh air smells.

3. **My nurses and care providers**. My nurses take great care of me all day and night long. Cedars hospital is a great hospital.

4. **My mom**, of course, who is my angel.

5. **Water**. I have never drank so much water in my life. Water is my life line from now on.

6. **Modern medicine.**

7. **All of you**. My friends and family who continually support me.

8. **My children**. This is obvious, but I will say it again. I love my kids so much. As they tell me, to the moon and back and 50 million billion times around!

9. **The stranger who made me smile today**. As I was walking around the floor with my head down I passed an elderly man. He smiled at me and said, "Good Luck, you're looking better."

10. **Life**. I am happy to be alive. I am still alive! That is the thing I am most grateful for!

On the next page, write 10 things that you are grateful for today.

"Acknowledging the good that you already have in your life is the foundation for all abundance." - Eckhart Tolle

Today, I am grateful for …

1. _____

2. _____

3. _____

4. _____

5. _____

6. _____

7. _____

8. _____

9. _____

10. _____

"Today I choose to live with gratitude for the love that fills my heart, the peace that rests within my spirit, and the voice of hope that says all things are possible." — Anonymous

Journal Time

Writing is healing and helps you connect with your own inner light source.

Here are my favorite journal prompts you can dive into to help you process all of the transformation and healing you're facing right now. In time, you will just put pen to paper (or fingers to keyboard) and begin to pour out your feelings, thoughts, fears, and dreams.

It's all about practice and not about perfection. Just show up for yourself. It's a beautiful demonstration of self-love!

What brings joy to your life? _____

_____

What is it that you've always wanted to do or be, but have been too afraid to try?

_____

_____

What are your fears? _____

_____

What makes you angry? _____

_____

What is the silver lining, the blessing, that cancer has brought to you? (I always tell people cancer saved my life because I wasn't living the life I dreamed of like I am now.)

_____

_____

In my bright future, I see … _____

_____

If I was able to write *my* ending to the story, it would go like this:

Start with the prompt, "Once upon a time ...." and write it all down. You may need to grab a couple more pieces of paper to continue if you have a lot to say!

_____

_____

_____

_____

_____

_____

Self-Forgiveness

We all have something inside of us we need to forgive ourselves for. What is it for you?

The time has come to forgive myself for _____

_____

If I had known better, I would have _____

_____

What do you regret? (I can share mine. I was living my life trying to impress others rather than living for myself. Today, I work hard on loving myself and my body and not being so self-critical.)

_____

_____

I want to make amends to my body, mind, and spirit for _____

_____

The valuable lessons I've learned from my mistakes are _____

_____

What is the one thing about your body you wish you could love and accept more? _____

_____

My Spiritual Support
Journey With Cancer

Before cancer, I didn't consider myself a spiritual person. As a child, I wondered why God gave me cancer and why he let my father die. In my heart I knew there was a higher power watching over me; I could feel it. Still, I was angry at God! How could he let such bad things happen to me at just four years old? Why did he make my family's life so hard? Now, I realize that all of those struggles gave me the strength I have today.

After I was diagnosed with cancer again, my biggest fear was dying and leaving behind my children. What would happen to them when I was gone?

I was in a constant state of anxiety and worry. I knew this was not the right state of mind to be in when you're trying to heal from cancer! At that point I was willing to try anything. I mean, *anything*!

My First Experience With a Healer

Before my big debulking surgery (when they took out as much of the tumor cells as possible), I drove alone to San Diego to meet an energy healer that I kept hearing about. I had no information on this man. My friend Kathy just said, he can help you. At that moment I was willing to try anything to get rid of my cancer. I just wanted it out of my body!

Once I arrived in San Diego, I drove down this alley and saw a sign that said, "Come in this gate for Steve." I have to be honest, I had no idea what to expect and I was a little skeptical when I walked through the gate.

Steve introduced himself and asked what was going on. Immediately, I burst into tears and couldn't talk. I had so much emotion and pain built up in me. I told him that I'm having a lot of anxiety because I just found out I have cancer AGAIN and I have a lot of anger. I mentioned how much guilt I was holding onto about my dad's suicide from my childhood. It was so crazy that all this past stuff was coming up for me.

Do you find trauma or fears from your past coming up now, during your cancer recovery? If you do, that's totally normal and it's a part of the healing process. Write down those memories and journal about all of your feelings, even the negative ones. This is a good time to begin healing old wounds so you can emerge from your recovery into a new life. A part of rebuilding yourself and moving forward is letting go of all the past, old stuff that doesn't serve you anymore.

Then the words, "I'm afraid to die," flowed out with my tears.

Steve started the session: first he put his hand on my belly for a few minutes. He just held still. I immediately started to feel heat radiate off his hands. It took maybe all of two minutes to feel this.

He said, "Oh Emilee, your energy lines are about to burst, you have so much toxic energy and waste in you." Then he said, "Your body can't handle any more stress in your life." Steve told me I would probably die of anger and stress before I died of cancer, that's how toxic I was. I read somewhere that, *"cancer eats toxins"* and this felt true to me. My body was so toxic that it was feeding the cancer and helping it grow.

Steve told me that he was going to do a technique with me that was going to separate my soul from my body. He explained that I would be flying over clouds (and he would be with me) and that I might see some colors. I remember him saying that the color violet is the ultimate healer.

"Ok? Kinda weird, but I'll go with it," I thought to myself. Steve began to brush my hair in a very specific pattern. He turned my head to the side and brushed up on my scalp very firmly, then he flipped my head to the other side and did the same thing. I thought, "awwww, this feels so good." This must be what it is like to be a cat or a dog who gets scratched and petted all day.

Then, Steve put oil onto my scalp and face. He started to massage very intensely. I was thinking about meeting my friend Trish after this and thought, "I hope he doesn't mess up my hair too much."

Next, Steve started tapping on my forehead, and then all over my head, it was like he was a little kid having fun playing the drums. It was very relaxing and I figured out why he was doing that. He was putting me into a relaxed, almost trance like state before he began what he was about to do.

Before I tell you the rest, you must know that I had never been to a healer. I didn't know what to expect. I had no idea about the power of energy.

The journey began ...

First I heard zen-full music.

"Quiet your my mind. You must think about nothing," Steve whispered.

I felt I was dreaming. My mind wouldn't quiet down. I was thinking about having a glass of wine with Trish and Russell afterwards, what I wanted to eat for dinner. All I could do was think about food, unable to quiet my mind and relax.

"Emilee, you must think about nothing and take a nap because you are so tired from your lack of sleep," is what I told myself. "Just go to sleep."

So, I did. I began to relax. I could feel the weight of my shoulders moving away from my ears, my collar bones began to broaden and my ribs became more relaxed. I could start to feel my breath becoming steady and smooth. I started to breathe in for four counts and then out for four counts. Just like I do in my yoga and Pilates practice. I thought a few more times to myself about what would happen if I opened my eyes. I asked myself, "am I wasting my time and money?" So many thoughts crossed my mind.

Steve placed his hands, more like his fingertips, onto the base of my skull. He held his hands there for what felt like two hours. It seemed like nothing was happening for awhile. Still nothing and I was getting frustrated because I took off work and drove four hours to see this guy.

Then all of a sudden, FLASH of blue! I thought to myself, was that really a flash of blue? The color was in the shape of a cloud. Then, another FLASH of blue, then green and back to blue again. This kept happening and then suddenly Steve jerked; it felt more like an abrupt jolt. It was like lightening had just passed through him and I felt a sudden shift in my energy.

I saw violet diamonds, blue clouds, green flashes and this kept going on and on. I had a big smile inside my body. If you have ever had surgery, it was almost that same feeling you get when the anesthesiologist says, "its time," and they take you to the operating room to give you the happy drink before you check out. There is a brief moment before you are totally out during surgery where everything turns white and is so peaceful.

I had never experienced anything like this. It was as if I just felt myself die. My biggest fear was confronted and it was beautiful on the other side. I felt my body go limp. For a moment in time, I felt nothing and heard nothing. I have never felt silence or peace ever like this. I was surrounded by a bright white light. That is the only color I saw. It all happened so fast. I wanted to stay longer, but my body was flooded with emotions. I began to cry almost uncontrollably, and within a few seconds I was back.

When I came back to normal consciousness I was in a blissful state. I wasn't afraid anymore. It was as if all of my anxieties and worries disappeared. I had a new sense of faith. I really believed that I was going to be OK, and if I wasn't, that was OK too. I wasn't afraid to die anymore which was my biggest fear since I was four years old because I almost died of cancer. Losing my dad to suicide at such a young age really scarred me too. What I experienced with Steve was peaceful and beautiful. It helped me process my cancer journey in a whole new way. I became more open to alternative healing methods.

I believe this was the experience that jumpstarted my body's healing process, even before the chemo and surgery.

Healing begins from the inside out. First you have to let go of old fear, anger and worries that don't serve you anymore.

After the session ended, I asked Steve, "What just happened? It felt like I just died for a moment."

He replied, "You did Emilee, for a brief moment. I detached your soul from your body. I took you to the other side," he said. Steve was healing me by performing a soul retrieval. A soul retrieval is used by energy healers and shamans to help people who have had major traumas in their lives: major operations, loss of loved ones, divorce and disease like cancer can all contribute to what shamans call a *loss of soul*.

Steve explained that as we were flying along we hit a wall. A BIG WALL. That's when Steve jolted. He shared that doesn't normally happen to him. He had to try extra hard to separate my body from my soul to take me to the other side. I know this sounds unreal, but it happened! And, I was completely skeptical.

Steve's feedback from our session was powerful: *"When we hit that wall it's because someone or something is holding you back. You are not ready to die. You were fighting me."*

I know now who that someone was – it was me! I had been fighting myself all of my life. I had been my biggest critic and my own worst enemy.

The soul retrieval was what I needed because I had completely lost myself. In order to become the hero of my own life, and teach others how to do the same, I had to finally rediscover who I was at the core of my being. I looked at this as a fresh start to create my new life.

After this experience, I embraced any and all forms of healing so I could truly live with peace, hope and joy.

Steve also said, "You're stronger than you've ever been. I can feel a shift in your energy." I also felt that.

This experience gave me the courage and hope to continue on even when I wanted to give up.

At the end of the session, he told me my entire right side needed more compassion.

Today, I send my body compassion every day. Do you? If not, today is the day. I say it out loud.

Repeat after me while placing your hands over your heart:

I send you love and compassion.
I send you love and compassion.
I send you love and compassion.

This has become the mantra I say to myself each day. You can do this too and notice how much more peaceful you feel.

Lastly, Steve told me I needed to conserve all my energy to fight this cancer. Anything toxic in my life had to be released. "Free up space for more stuff that will come …stuff will always come," he said, "and you just need to learn to let it go!"

Those words honestly have been the greatest gift I have been given.

What can you let go of so that you can receive more of what you want and need in your life?

Fear? Anger? Resentment? Guilt? Shame?

We all have something. What is it for you?

Now you have more space for what you truly deserve: Love, compassion, joy and forgiveness.

You matter.

Meeting With The Shaman

I was beginning to believe in miracles and the power of positive thinking and energy healing.

After the extraordinary healing session with Steve, I was introduced to another man who has become one of my dearest friends, Shaman Jon.

Jon, who drove down from Big Sur, California, arrived at my door. My dog Winston, who we all called Winston the Wonder Dog, was a little unsure of him at first. Winston, a small white bichon poodle, took care of me and protected me throughout my whole struggle with cancer.

When Jon got on the floor and started talking to Winston, my normally *ferocious* guard dog suddenly became calm. Winston jumped on his lap and sat with Jon the entire time he was talking to me. Normally Winston would be all over me. From that moment, I knew this man had a special touch. I had never seen my dog like this. It was hilarious; he was rolling over on his back for him to be petted and it was almost as if Winston was needing some healing from his past too.

Jon opened up his bag of "stuff." I saw rattles, blankets, eagle feathers, crystals and much more. John started off with an introduction of what he did and explained about our Karma and ancestors.

I had so many questions! I asked him the same questions so many other cancer patients ask: "Why me?" I asked him why I couldn't get over my past anger. He smiled and said, *"it's all stuff we are going to work on, but you are on your way. A lot of this shit in life that we are given comes from our ancestors. It's their unfinished business that we have to deal with."*

Jon told me he was going to perform a soul retrieval. He explained that the soul retrieval brings back parts of the lost soul as well as the passion and the gifts that those parts hold for you. The objective of a soul retrieval is to make you whole again; it changes the myths or beliefs that are creating the same experiences over and over again.

He began to brush a feather up and down my body with a very light touch. I closed my eyes and surrendered to the healing. I had no idea if it was working at that time, but looking back now I can tell you that something inside of me changed forever. It was one of the first times in my life that I felt safe and allowed myself to fully open up, especially to a stranger. I had seen psychologists before, but this was different. Maybe it was a sense of trust and compassion that I have never felt before from anyone. I knew this guy wasn't judging me.

I shared my entire life story with him, the good and the bad, and he didn't think I was crazy and he didn't shame me. He said, "I have been down a similar path, you are not alone." Honestly, those words changed my life. To know that I was not going to be alone on this journey, when I felt so isolated and alone, is the reason I am alive today. Shaman Jon gave me hope and helped me find my spirit to live again.

This is why I'm sharing my stories with you. I don't want you to feel alone, like I did. Sometimes all we have to hang on to is hope.

I was struggling with anxiety, angry feelings and paranoia about going out in public. Jon taught me how to push away negative energy and people to protect my own health. These are the keys to cancer recovery: self-love, self-respect and self-care. Some people may call it selfish, but it is necessary to survive. It's a survival skill that helped me save my life. It's critical that you put yourself first during this time.

When you surround yourself by other people who have good energy you will feel more positive. Haven't you ever been around someone so negative they just sucked the life out of you? It feels like they absorb all of your energy. This is the energy you do not want to have. You want high vibrational, positive energy around you. When you are positive, you attract good things. For me, it was survival. I was attracting life, breath and all good things to come.

Jon placed a colorful blanket on my bed and then put stones, feathers, crystals, and a little pouch on it. He said, "pick the stones that you feel connected with." I picked five stones, but the one I was really drawn to was a beautiful, shimmering crystal. I had heard that crystals had healing powers and kept them in my home because they added beauty. My kids collected crystals! Having crystals around me still gives me a sense of protection. I highly recommend getting some crystals for yourself. I love heart-shaped ones, but pick ones that appeal to you the most. Pink-colored rose quartz is a great one to keep around you: it enhances feelings of happiness and self-love.

I laid down on my bed as he placed a stone on my forehead, throat, heart-chakra in the center of my chest, and all the way down the midline of my body.

Jon picked up a bottle that he would sip out of that contained some healing herbs in it. He would chant, take a swig and then blow it in the air over me. I thought that was weird at first, but all I really wanted was to be healed so I stayed open minded. At some point, I felt my body get a little hot. I couldn't hold back the tears or the pain any longer. My tears started to fall like Niagara Falls. I had been afraid to allow myself to cry since childhood because I thought it meant that you were showing weakness. I wanted to be strong, especially for my mother when I was young. I was worried that my tears would upset her and cause her to worry.

At the end of the session he asked me what I saw in his eyes. I said, "focus and determination."

YES! **What you focus on you get.**

Jon said, "I see a lot of sparkling and shimmering in your eyes."

He also reminded me that I have the birthright to be on this planet, and that now it's my time to shine.

After he told me this, I used this mantra daily to help me get through the difficult days ahead:

This is my time to shine!

Even if you don't feel it right now, it's your time to shine too. By saying this mantra, you are changing your thought patterns. We are all shining miracles. I believe in you.

After our session, Jon wrote this to me:

"For you Emilee,

When I did the work with you, I found that you had been holding energy and patterns of all six painful experiences from several lifetimes, as well as that of your DNA ancestors.

When we cleared each and every chakra of the old wounds, and performed the death and rebirth, you let go of your ancestor's wounds.

We also did the destiny retrieval to boost the patterns of your greatness as a Medicine Woman. So now all of your wounds and struggles have become your gifts and medicine to others.

As now in this life, since the universe will make your new story right, others will respect you and see you as this great, powerful, and benevolent Medicine Woman/ Shaman, as you will own and see yourself. You will receive unconditional love and support from men and women, and everything you have to do on the mind and body levels will be much easier and more effective. Your health and vitality, strength and suppleness will improve in every way.

You have the support of all of the forces of nature and shamanic lineages within you to assist you unconditionally."

I want to pass onto you the unconditional love and support I received from these healers.

The lesson from these two stories that I want you to walk away with is this: whatever you're holding onto right now: anger, fear, resentment, stress, sadness. Get it out! Release it from your mind, body and soul.

Holding onto these toxic emotions can be dangerous and deadly.

Create Your Own Team of Healers

I wanted to share my experience with the energy healing of Steve and Jon the Shaman, to inspire you to look outside of traditional treatments for cancer. You can integrate alternative forms of healing with Western medicine for great results. Every week, I saw both an acupuncturist, and a Chinese doctor who prescribed a tea of medicinal herbs (that frankly tasted and smelled awful).

If you have never tried any of these therapies and aren't sure where to find the best practitioners in your area, try asking your local cancer center or do a Google search.

Who do you want on your dream team of healers?

Make a list of the healers you and your body need.

Some examples: massage, acupuncture, Chinese medicine, nutritionist, herbalist, Pilates, yoga, tapping, spiritual community centers, energy healers, reiki, psychologists, support groups.

You can't and you shouldn't do this alone.

Exercise Tips for When You Have an Ostomy

If you haven't had ostomy surgery you can skip over this chapter and move on.

If you have, please continue reading because I wish someone would have told me what I'm about to tell you!

There is so much I want to share from my own experience of having an ileostomy, but I don't want to overwhelm you at a time like this, while you're recovering and healing from cancer. What you need the most right now is to feel calm and have peace of mind.

I hope this chapter can help you take it easy on yourself after all that you've been through.

After you've had ostomy surgery, I'm not going to lie and tell you that your life will go back to normal right away. Your body will feel different and you will feel different about your body. It's normal to get down and feel depressed. When you do, the best medicine is to get outside and go for a walk or share your feelings with a support group. Clear your head. Walking always made me feel better. Even if it was only two houses away from mine, which took five minutes to do. I walked as slow as a turtle.

Don't judge or criticize yourself; just get up and move your body. That is the best medicine.

Shortly after having my ileostomy surgery, I Googled "exercises to do with a new ileostomy," and could not find much except a lot of contradictory information!

Most stuff I read online said, *"No weights, no ab workouts, no running."* One site said to go back to your normal routine, which was terrible advice–THE WORST.

DO NOT jump back into the old routine you did before the ostomy surgery too soon!

Even though I had been a movement educator, Pilates and yoga instructor for 17 years, I had to start all over. I wanted to figure out a way to move my body. I needed to get back to my studio and work, since I was a single mom going through a divorce and raising three kids.

Of course, I had found certain limitations that I worked through, and that is why I want to help you.

How to Begin a New Way of Exercising

If you're reading this book in the hospital, begin with *Phase 1: Exercises in the Hospital.* Seems logical, right?

If you're home recovering from your ostomy surgery, begin by opening up to the chapter titled, *Phase 2: Recovery at Home.*

All of these exercises that begin in bed might look simple to somebody who hasn't been put through the wringer like you. But trust me, they are perfect for helping you rehabilitate your whole body.

These exercises start off nice and gentle in bed. You are on your back a lot during recovery, so I included some that you can do lying on your side. These will help strengthen your hips for walking. You need to move your body and get the blood flowing, even while resting and recovering in your bed.

Side note: your body and midsection, where your incision and ostomy is, will love you for doing the gentle bridge in bed where you prop your hips up with pillows. It's a nice stretch across your lower pelvis and back. (You can take a peek at that stretch right now in *Phase 2.*)

Believe me, at some point, you will get sick of sitting on the couch and watching TV, or lying in bed in the same old boring positions. The first two phases of this book contain simple exercises that you can do in bed or in a chair. They will keep you focused and motivated toward healing and getting your body back.

That is your goal, right? Sitting around will not get you those results.

This book was created with you in mind. I know you can get up and move your body, even for five minutes. I believe in you! I've been in your shoes and I know at times it will be hard to get moving. Do your best and remind yourself that *movement is medicine.*

We all recover at different rates and have different levels of pain tolerance. **Listen to your body and if you feel pain, stop.** It may mean that your body isn't ready to do that particular exercise yet.

Pain is a signal that something isn't happy in your body. Move on to the next exercise until you find one that feels good. And if you get frustrated, come back and try another day, but don't give up. Never give up.

Remind yourself that it's about progress, not perfection. This is not a competition to see who can heal from cancer the fastest!

Try out one or two of the many stretches in the *Stretch* chapter each day. A little stretch can go a long way!

The primary goal of this book is to help you get your deep core muscles strong so that you can go back to doing any form of exercise you really love, safely and without pain.

When you begin to exercise—or let's just say move your body, because it doesn't seem like exercise in the beginning—you may have to modify some stuff. But in reality, anytime you move your body, you are doing a form of exercise. **Think of each small movement as medicine for your body.**

After you complete Phase 1 and 2, check out the chapter *All About Your Core*. It will give you the lowdown on the important muscle groups that support so much of your basic, day-to-day activities (for example, sitting down and standing up).

When you're feeling stronger, progress to Phase 4 and 5, where you will learn balance and strengthening exercises.

Exercise Tips

- Move as slow as molasses. The best advice I can give you is this: *please* do not push or move at a fast pace when doing abdominal work. This can pull on the insides (intestines) and cause discomfort, tears, strains, or even worse, a hernia. Slower movements take more control and focus.
- When exercising, tuck your bag into your underwear or into your yoga pants. I could not live without high-waisted yoga pants. You can also wear snug biking shorts. This makes your stoma and pouching system feel more secure.
- Order yourself an ostomy belt–you can try one brand called the Stealth Belt (www.stealthbelt.com). I've heard nothing but good things about them!
- Make sure that you empty your pouch before exercising.
- Always have an extra change of clothes and supplies on hand.
- Hydrate. Drink a lot of water!
- If you shower after exercising, try using a hair dryer on the lowest setting to dry the back of your pouching system.

Don't sweat it! You will get the hang of this. If you're anything like I was after surgery, you're probably afraid you will hurt yourself when you exercise. If you follow this guidebook closely, you will safely restore your strength from the inside out.

You can do more than you think you can! Respect your body and remember to do everything in this book *slowly*.

One woman in my **Cancer Core Recovery® Program** had a hernia, and she was able to do all of the exercises pain free. Each individual is unique, so always listen to your body, and make sure you get medical clearance from your doctor if you have a hernia.

Remember, there is no rush. Healing is a process.

My Tips for Dealing with Your New Ostomy

- Practice changing your ostomy bag before surgery, if possible. The doctor can provide you with a kit that includes an instructional DVD and a "fake" stoma–it's meant to be helpful and educational. I opened the kit, put on the DVD, and walked away. I was still in denial that all of this was happening to me. That was mistake #1. Watch the video, even if you don't want to.
- The first few times you watch the video about changing your ostomy bag, do it by yourself so you can focus and even take notes. Mistake #2: I had my friends over to watch the video with me. My friends started to cry, which made me feel even worse. I didn't want to watch it after that. Your friends are not going to be there changing your new ostomy for you, so don't invite them to the video premiere! In the end, you may find yourself taking care of your friends' feelings and emotions instead of your own. This is the time when you need to focus on yourself and be a little selfish. *This is self-care.*
- Slow down. Changing your ostomy can take from thirty to forty minutes in the beginning because it's overwhelming and new.
- Be gentle as you clean around your stoma. If you don't, you can get blisters and irritated skin like I did, and that is no fun.
- Use a heating pad, or heat up your wafer and rings in your hands. If you don't have a heating pad, use the second-best thing like your car seat warmer, if you're on the go.
- Always carry an extra trash bag or ziplock bag and always have extra supplies on you (especially scissors).
- Always carry extra clothes, washcloths and small trash bags with you–I had more than one bag leak in my car. Messy! Having an extra

set of clean clothes and a plastic bag to put the soiled ones in saved the day!

- Empty your pouch or bag anywhere from five to eight times a day. If you wait too long to empty your pouch, it can pull on your stoma and be very uncomfortable.

How to Calmly Change Your Ostomy Bag

The first bag change at home may freak you out a little. It's inevitable. What I want to share with you next is how I got through the initial panic and made it to the other side, by asking for help.

You do not have to do this alone. Get all the help you can from the nurses while you're in the hospital. When you get home and need assistance, call on your rep from the medical device company. That's what I did, and it really saved the day!

I'd like to share a few highlights and the steps the nice man on the phone led me through as I changed my ostomy for the first time.

I said to him, *"I think I'm dying."*

First thing he said was, *"It is messy, but you will not die."* I was in full-on crisis mode, and this man calmly talked me down. He should have received the Hero of the Year Award in my eyes.

Here are the instructions he gave me, and I want to share them with you so you don't have to panic like I did.

Get your **washcloths** handy and near your sink. Remove your pouch, and then remove all of the adhesive with the no-sting universal remover wipe (or medical adhesive remover). This includes the ring and anything sticky around it. Remove *all* of it!

Then, heat up a warm washcloth and place it on your stoma with some gentle pressure. This calms down the activity of the digestive fluids coming out, and it feels good. The warmth also helps to calm your nervous system.

There are moments where your stoma feels like lava is flowing out of you and you feel like it's never going to stop. The craziest part of this is that you have zero control over how much or when your body will excrete these fluids. Your stoma has no shut-off valve. Sometimes I went through four or five washcloths at a time. I recommend buying some cheap washcloths because you will ruin your nice ones.

Once the flow of output has calmed down and you feel like it's a good time, take another dry washcloth and dab or gently pat your skin around the stoma. At the same time, hold the washcloth on your stoma (with some gentle pressure). Use this time to heat up your products (wafer and rings).

This was the process I learned, and this is what ended up working best for me. Of course, it's all trial and error, and there is no one right way.

I plugged in a heating pad and set the two small rings and wafer on the heating pad to warm them up. This helps them mold to your skin better and secure the seal, preventing a leak.

During this time, I would get my small, sharp scissors and guesstimate the size of the hole I needed to cut in order for it to fit perfectly over my stoma. First, I would cut a hole and place it over my stoma. If it looked too small, then I would cut some more. There really is no easy way. It's a cut-and-go process. This was the hardest part for me. I was terrible at getting the right size hole, but eventually, once my stoma shrank and became more consistent, I knew the approximate size I could cut every time.

Once your skin and the area around your stoma are cleaned and dry, it's time to quickly put on the ring and wafer. You don't have long until the next round of output starts flowing from your stoma. Take the ostomy barrier paste (if you are using paste) and carefully line the area around your stoma. It will even out the skin surface around your stoma. The paste comes in a tube that looks like toothpaste. It provides a barrier between your skin and stoma. It also helps to make a better seal with your ostomy bag and prevents leaks.

Once the paste is on, quickly untie the wrapper from the ring and mold it over your stoma.

Look to make sure there are no areas where the liquid or fluid can leak out onto your skin. This is important; otherwise, the liquid (digestive contents) will burn you. It's like acid sitting on your skin. I know the feeling well because it happened to me and I got painful blisters that bled.

Stay on top of cleaning yourself. If you get blisters or irritation, there is a great powder that you can use to absorb excess moisture from your skin. Keep the powder minimal if you are going to use it. Too much powder can weaken the seal. You want a sticky surface for your ring and bag to attach to.

There basically is a product for everything, but I learned that less is better!

I promise it will get easier every time you change your bag. It will become simpler as you get your new routine down.

You've got this.

Phase 1: Recovery in the Hospital

Welcome to Phase 1! You're still in the hospital, recovering in your bed and coming out of the fog, because you're still on all those medications and painkillers.

The exercises in this guide were designed for and inspired by individuals who have had abdominal and ostomy surgeries.

These exercises are great for any recovery, but you will hear me specifically reference the abdomen a lot!

If you have had breast surgery, skip the arm exercises until you have clearance from your doctor or can modify appropriately for your comfort and safety.

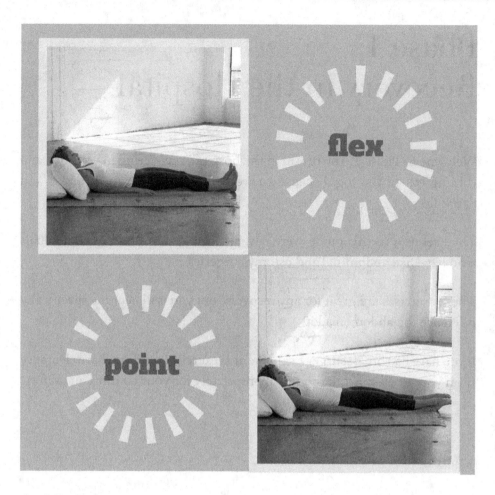

Ankle Pumps

Lie in bed and simply flex and point your feet to wake them up.

You can do it slowly or briskly.

This stimulates blood flow. Blood clots are a big concern if you're in bed for too long, so simple moves like these will help move blood throughout your body.

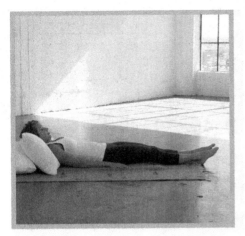

Leg Slides

This movement stimulates blood flow.

Lie on your back with straight legs.

Breathe in and exhale as you slowly slide your right leg up to bend your knee.

Breathe in and exhale as you slide your leg back to start position.

Start with ten to twenty repetitions on each leg.

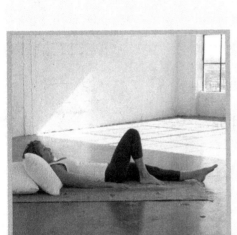

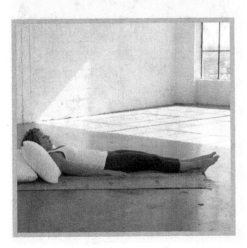

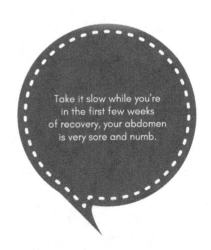

Take it slow while you're in the first few weeks of recovery, your abdomen is very sore and numb.

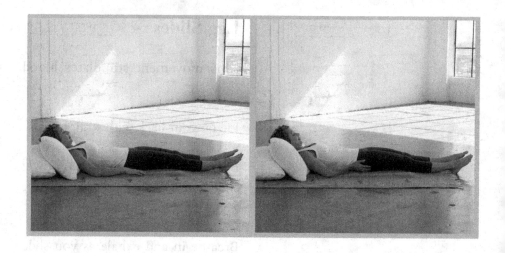

Butt Squeezes

It's as simple as it sounds. Squeeze your butt!

This can be done lying down or standing.

Simply squeeze and release.

Repeat twenty times.

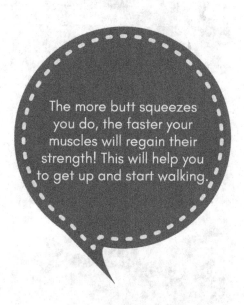

The more butt squeezes you do, the faster your muscles will regain their strength! This will help you to get up and start walking.

Knee Fallout

Lie on your back. Bend your knees with your feet flat on the bed.

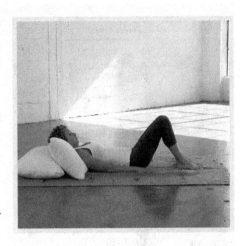

Slowly let one leg fall to the side while keeping the opposite hip down.

Return to the center.

Repeat this action ten times as a slow movement.

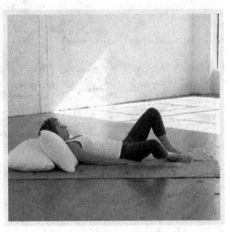

Repeat on other side. You can also stay with your leg open to the side for a longer stretch.

Gently stretch and relax.

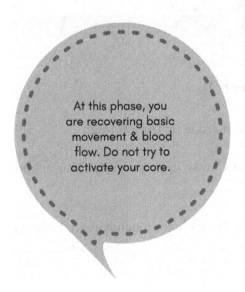

At this phase, you are recovering basic movement & blood flow. Do not try to activate your core.

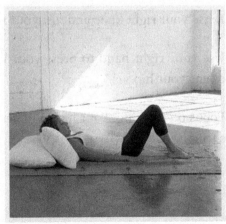

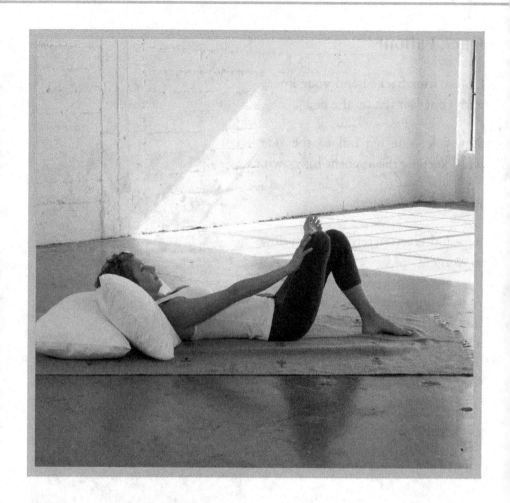

Simple Figure Four Hip Stretch

Raise your right knee and rest your right ankle on the left thigh.

Use your right hand to press your knee away from your hip. This action opens your hip.

Focus on relaxing. Your hips will get tight from too much lying in bed and sitting!

Stretch!

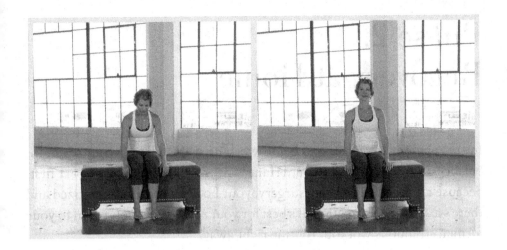

Sit Tall

Even though you feel very weak at this point, I want you to practice sitting tall and breathing.

I am assuming you are still hooked up to your IV cart and have tubes hanging off of you.

Slowly lift your chest and hold your body upright in a sitting tall posture. I understand—it's painful.

You will feel scar tissue pulling on the inside. This is normal. It's good to move through this slowly.

With each breath, imagine that you are creating space inside your body. I'm proud of you! This is a huge step toward getting stronger!

> Imagine a fishhook under your breastbone pulling you up as you sit tall, opening up the front of your body.

Phase 2:
Recovery at Home

In this phase, you're going to begin working on rebuilding your strength, balance and flexibility. It is important to work on the flexibility part first, because after you've just had surgery, your body has been traumatized and there's a lot of inflammation. It's best for your recovery to not return to your former, strenuous workout routine right away.

Remember that you're on a healing journey. Take your time, have patience and give your body the love that it needs. Always respect and listen to your body.

We're going to begin this phase with easy exercises and stretches that you can do in your bed at home.

Simple Knee Lift

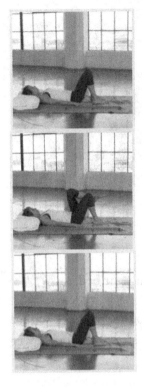

Lie in bed. Inhale and breathe slowly into your chest.

Exhale and slowly lift your right knee up toward your chest.

Hold for four slow counts, allowing the leg to feel heavy into your pelvis.

Exhale and slowly lower the leg, keeping your pelvis glued to the bed. Imagine your pelvis like a cement block. The only thing moving is your leg—slowly.

Repeat five to ten times in bed slowly and increase as you get stronger.

Think of your leg like a pumping system that helps pump and dump out the toxins.

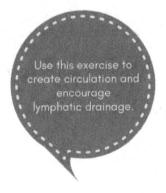

Use this exercise to create circulation and encourage lymphatic drainage.

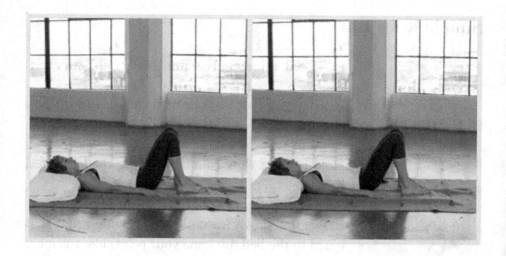

Pelvic Tilt

Lie down with your knees bent and feet resting flat on your bed.

Start with a slow inhale, then exhale and gently rock your pelvis back so that your lower back sinks into the bed. You will feel a nice stretch in your lower back.

Stay for a few breaths and enjoy the stretch.

Slowly rock back to start position.

Repeat as many times as your body craves it.

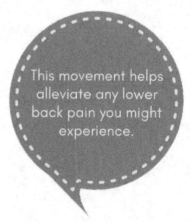

This movement helps alleviate any lower back pain you might experience.

Belly Stretch with Pillow under Hips

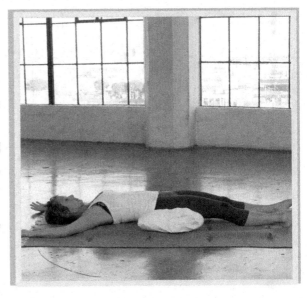

Lift up your hips and place a pillow under your pelvis.

Stretch your legs out. This is my favorite movement to help stretch your tummy and scar tissue.

Inhale; breathe into your belly. Visualize with each inhalation that you are gently stretching your scar tissue, and tell yourself that soon you will be back on your feet.

Exhale and relax.

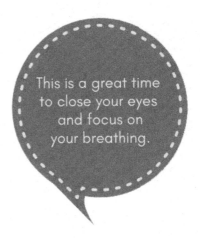

This is a great time to close your eyes and focus on your breathing.

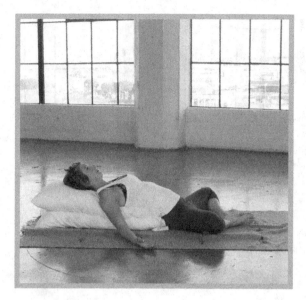

Supported Reclining Frog

This can be done in your bed or on the floor. Place a few pillows lengthwise behind your back. If your head hangs back, support it with another pillow.

Lie back and relax into the pillows. Allow your legs to slowly fall open to either side (like frog legs).

Breathe into the abdomen, relaxing your abdomen and pelvis. With each breath, let go of any tension you are holding onto.

Stay for up to three to five minutes.

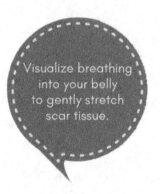

Visualize breathing into your belly to gently stretch scar tissue.

Child's Pose in Bed

If you are able, get onto your knees and curl yourself into a ball-like position, as shown in the picture. This is another great pose to help relax your back.

Stretch your arms forward in bed and feel the stretch through your entire body.

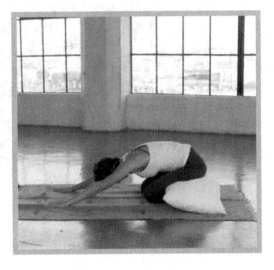

Your inner thighs will most likely be tight post-surgery, so relax your legs open to a comfortable position where you can rest your torso between your legs.

Take time to breathe and relax.

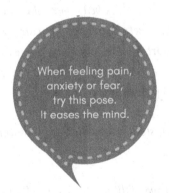

When feeling pain, anxiety or fear, try this pose. It eases the mind.

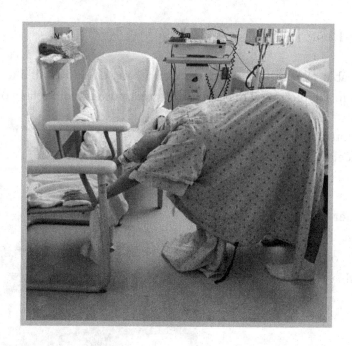

Before we move on to the next exercise, I want to tell you a story.

So, you have to laugh at this. My nurse forced me out of my bed, even when I didn't want to get up. She said it was time to change the sheets. I dreaded her coming in to do this because it meant that I had to put out effort to move my body. Some days, I was too afraid to move because the pain was off the charts. After I got out of bed and into my chair, I noticed that I actually started to feel better.

One day, I carefully placed my hands on the chair, stood up, turned around, and did a modified downward dog stretch. It felt so good.

Of course the nurse ran over to me and thought I was falling, but I said, "I'm okay. I'm doing yoga. I'm stretching my legs and belly."

By this point, I had lost any flexibly I ever had. I was starting from the very beginning.

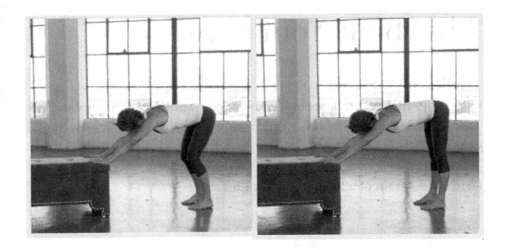

Downward Dog

Place your hands on the bed and step your legs back with your feet apart.

Press your hands into your bed, bend your knees slightly, and feel a good stretch in the back of your legs. Try to keep your heels down if possible.

As your legs get more flexible, try to straighten them more.

Relax and breathe in this position for thirty to sixty seconds.

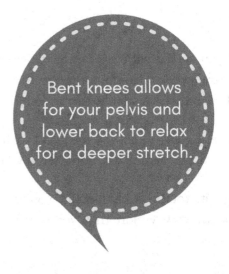

Bent knees allows for your pelvis and lower back to relax for a deeper stretch.

All About Your Core

First things first: let's talk about what your core really is. No, it's not the "six pack" muscles that many of us think we're supposed to possess to have a strong core.

Here is a diagram of what makes up your core.

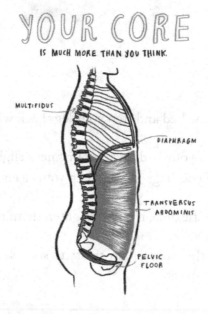

As you can see in the diagram above, the muscles that make up the core include the transverse abdominis, the multifidus, the pelvic floor, and the diaphragm. These muscles work together to stabilize the spine and pelvic girdle.

I'm not going to get too technical with you, because I'm sure you've had it with all the medical terms thrown at you after you got diagnosed with cancer.

I get it. You probably feel like you've just graduated from medical school. You know way more than you ever wanted to about the human body. But

I know you can handle learning about one more muscle. It's a muscle that we'll stretch a lot in this program.

It's called the psoas. After surgery, especially in your abdomen and pelvis, this muscle feels tight, so we will stretch it gently. Stretching the psoas will help you with your posture as well as the back pain you may have experienced with surgery.

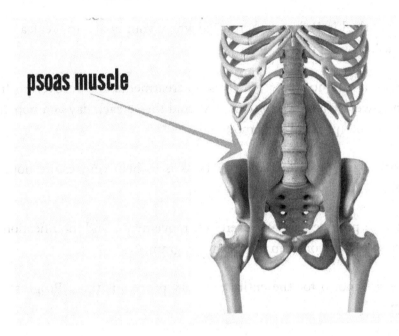

psoas muscle

Laura Horn, Physical Therapist specializing in female pelvic conditions, has this to say about the importance of the core muscles: During your daily activities, the core muscles work at low levels at all times and increase their activation before a movement occurs. In other words, they tighten when you roll out of bed in the morning and as you stand from a chair. These muscles tighten before you reach into the fridge for that quart of almond milk, and they tighten before you lift your organic produce from your car.

All of these muscles should activate and work together to support each other, but most importantly, they need to support your body so that you don't suffer from back and pelvic pain.

I'd love nothing more than for you to put all of this pain behind you and rebuild your body so that you can get back on your feet, take back your life, and put this stupid cancer behind you.

I believe in you! Whenever you feel like giving up or start to lose hope, think of me jumping up and down with my pom-poms cheering you on. (Yep, I was a cheerleader in high school! I love encouraging people. It's just who I am.)

This is not the kind of workout routine where your goal is to break a sweat. This is a "thrival" program.

While we are fighting for our lives on treatments and recovering from surgeries, we are just trying to survive and thrive each day and hopefully get out of pain (physical and emotional).

The goal of my programs and this book is to help you restore hope for yourself.

I wanted to provide as many exercises, movements, and modifications as possible so that anyone can follow my program.

My favorite motto for the entire recovery process is this: "Progress, not perfection."

Remind yourself of this often.

About Breathing

Have you ever watched a jellyfish swim? I love watching them at the aquarium with my kids.

They look so peaceful.

I had my illustrator, Joya, draw this jellyfish for you because I often visualize them while I move and breathe.

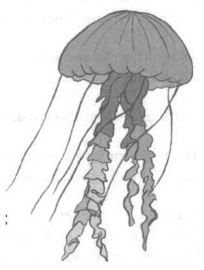

Jellyfish are strong (like you), but they are also graceful and move in a gentle way. This is how I want you to move; imagine you are a jellyfish!

BREATHE.

Slow. Gentle. Strong.

Breathing is so important!

Not only is the breath our life force, but it also helps to regulate our anxieties and fears.

Slowing down your breath will help you focus more on yourself, and that is what you need right now. One hundred percent full love and attention for *you*.

Here's a breathing visualization you can try out while you're doing the exercises in this book.

Imagine a jellyfish in the ocean. In order for it to move up to the surface of the water, it has to tighten up its body and use its strong tentacles to give it power.

Jellyfish are flexible and can change shape—just like us.

When you do each stretch and exercise, or even while getting up out of bed, use your breath and imagine you are a jellyfish moving through the sea. Move slowly and with intention. Take extra time to get where you want to go. You don't need to move through life so fast, right? Jellyfish are slow movers.

Enjoy each movement and learn to feel your body—and watch it get strong and graceful.

A little more about **The Physiology of Breathing**.

The diaphragm is an important muscle. It is your breathing muscle. It is also one of the four muscle groups that make up your core region.

Imagine your torso broken into upper (thoracic) and lower (abdominal) cavities. Later in this guide, I call them your upper core and your lower core. Your lower cavity contains your colon, bladder, kidneys, pancreas, stomach, liver, gall bladder, and more. Your thoracic or upper cavity contains your heart, lungs, and rib cage.

The important thing to know is that the diaphragm separates these two cavities.

Both of these cavities have the ability to change shape. You probably are most aware of the belly breath; that's because it's the most natural way to breathe. Think of babies: when they breathe in and out, you can see their abdomens expand with the inhalation and relax with the exhalation. This is the kind of breathing you will be doing for the first six to eight weeks of your recovery to relax your abdomen and pelvic floor region.

Try this. It's easy: take a deep breath into your abdomen and notice your belly stretch; then exhale and visualize your pelvis and abdomen beginning to relax.

Slowly inhale for four counts and feel your belly rise; then exhale for four counts and feel your belly relax. You may feel scar tissue inside breaking apart as you do this simple breath, and that is great! I did a lot of this breathing in my hospital bed and at home in recovery. Every time I lay back down after sitting or standing, it seemed like my abdomen and scar would tighten up again. The simple act of gentle breathing can help keep scar tissue from reforming.

Later, when we get into phase 3 and begin to rehabilitate your core, the breathing technique changes. You might wonder why.

When we begin to strengthen your core region, you want to avoid letting your abdomen bulge out. Instead, you want the abdomen to gently pull in and create a lifting up feeling inside your rib cage. This allows for a more supportive core.

Think of it as a lifting action, not a sucking-in action. If you let your belly hang out, there is no support for your back.

Just one more fun visual for you: think back to when you were a kid and maybe had a water balloon fight with your friends. You fill up the water balloons and then squeeze them really hard from the bottom, and you watch all the water move up and spread to the top. The top of the balloon expands, but the bottom, where you are squeezing and holding tight, doesn't bulge or move. Use this image as you're breathing when engaging your deep core muscles. As you breathe, move the oxygen up to your lungs, but keep your waist and midsection narrowed and engaged!

I know I spend a lot of time talking to you about breathing, but it's important.

Heck, breathing is more important in recovery because if you don't breathe, the anxiety kicks in and sometimes you might feel like you are having a panic attack.

Deep-breathe in and deep-breathe out—and wash your worries away!

Abdominal Self-Massage

Begin this at home after your stomach is healed and there are no open wounds.

Start by standing in front of a mirror.

This is an awesome time to say your daily affirmations: tell yourself how beautiful you are and how much gratitude you have for your body, even though you may not feel that way right now. One of my favorite affirmations is by *Crazy Sexy Cancer* author Kris Carr:

> In case you forget to remind yourself....
> Your butt is perfect.
> Your smile lights up the room.
> Your mind is insanely cool.
> You are way more than enough.
> And you are doing an amazing job at life.

Before, during, and after my cancer diagnosis, constipation was a daily problem in my life. It was actually my first symptom to being diagnosed with ovarian cancer.

Poop is one of my favorite subjects now. Cancer treatment, surgery, and especially chemotherapy can leave you feeling miserable and constipated. There is nothing worse than this.

Often after surgery and being on pain medications, your body and intestines get sluggish and slow down. **Constipation** is a *big* problem. **Drink** lots of water and walk to help this issue. Plus, this self-abdominal massage can really help get that poop moving again!

You can do this daily massage once you feel comfortable enough to touch your stomach. At first, the nerves are very sensitive around the entire abdomen.

Once your scar has healed and the doctor says it looks good and clears you, start the self-massage.

Start the colon massage and scar tissue releasing at the left lower quadrant of the abdomen—but first, take a look at the picture of the poop moving through the intestines below. Your massage imitates peristaltic movement of matter through the intestine.

Gently place both hands to start the self-massage. You should feel the massage, but it shouldn't hurt. Place one palm on top of the other palm. Find your left pelvic bone. Take your hands and place them on the bottom right side of your abdomen and massage up the bottom of your ribs. Then move across the bottom of your ribcage towards the left side, pressing gently. Now, move down the left side towards the bottom of your lower abdomen.

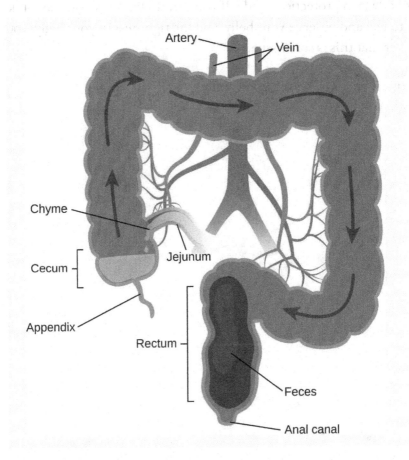

This covers your entire colon, and some places in between. I also recommend massaging around your navel, as this action massages the small intestines; just think of it like a circle. This can be done with lotion or not. I recommend lotion because it helps your dry and itchy skin while it's healing. Coconut oil is great!

During the self-massage, you might feel lumps and bumps inside. This can be scar tissue building up.

This self-massage will help stretch scar tissue in the surrounding abdomen. It's important to remember that it's not just your external scar you see that causes the belly tightness. It is all of the internal scar tissue fibers that are being built up inside and around the surrounding area.

Your body is in protection mode. If you can slow things down and take the time to feel and observe your belly, and the tightness in your belly, you will discover that this is scar tissue.

Scar tissue needs to be stretched *gently*.

Scar Stretch

Once the nerve pain goes away and you feel comfortable touching the area around your scar, or even on top of the scar (as long as there is no open wound and it is completely healed up), start moving your fingers down the scar.

Gently press in toward your abdomen and move the scar tissue around slowly. Remember, be gentle.

I noticed a lot of scar tissue around my naval and upper intestines, where my stoma was inserted. After my ostomy was reversed four months later, I noticed a large internal lump of scar tissue. Scar tissue can be *very painful*.

It's important to follow what feels right. I was comfortable massaging myself and always poking my fingers into my abdomen because I knew it would help me.

In the beginning of recovery, the more you can stand up and stretch your belly, the better.

Sometimes that can be enough movement and stretching for you that day.

Still, my favorite way to stretch my scar (because it's always tight) is to lie back over pillows, large stability balls, or anything that would stretch my belly.

Water Intake

Make sure to **drink** lots of water during your recovery!

Even though I'm sure you're tired of hearing about how much water you need, I can't emphasize this enough!

All those pain medications will back you up. You don't want to become dehydrated. If you have a new ostomy, dehydration happens quickly, so please make sure you drink up every day!

Also, if you're still on chemo, you probably already know this: you get dehydrated.

Have water next to your bed, in your purse, and in your car at all times.

Phase 3: Exercises to Strengthen Your Core

Phase 3 includes my unique core recovery exercises that were inspired by my ileostomy. The slow and small movements in this phase (using the stability balls) help activate and retrain your deep core muscles just enough to engage and strengthen them, without overdoing it.

You will be surprised at how small movements will be felt so deeply. There are no quick crunches or sit ups, just mindful movements to help you rebuild your core.

In this section, you're going to use props like small and large stability balls. The reason why I use these props is because it feels so much better on your back and it helps you to find your deep abdominal muscles without straining. And the last thing you want to do in your recovery is strain yourself or cause a hernia.

So, be patient, be kind and remember that all these moves that I teach you are very, very, very small; they may not look like a lot, but they are working deep inside your core.

Props You Will Need:

Order two 9-10 inch exercise stability balls for this phase, if you don't already own any. I get mine from Amazon and my two favorite companies are Merrithew and Overball.

How to Inflate Your Stability Balls:

First, stick the straw in the little hole, then blow the ball up. Don't over inflate the balls because they will be too firm. It takes about 4 big exhales!

As soon as you pull out the straw, stick in the plug. The ball should have a little squish to it.

Upper Core Exercises

In this series of exercises, timing and coordination are key.

All movements should be done in slow counts of four. Four counts to slowly lift. Four counts to hold in place. Four counts to slowly lower.

In the exercise instructions I mention to sink or press your feet into the floor a lot.

This is a very important action. I want you to imagine your feet as the foundation to these exercises. I know that sounds weird, but you will notice that when you sink your feet into the floor combined with squeezing the ball, you will notice your core activate on a much deeper level.

Upper Back Stretch

Place one ball under your upper mid-back, between your shoulder blades. The ball should not be in the lower back or neck. It should feel comfortable.

Place the second ball between your knees, and keep it engaged throughout the exercise.

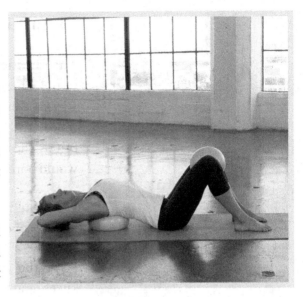

Interlace your fingers together and place them behind your head. Rest your head in your hands.

Open your chest, and lie back over the ball.

You will feel your belly stretch; it should feel good. Take a few breaths into your abdomen and allow yourself to relax.

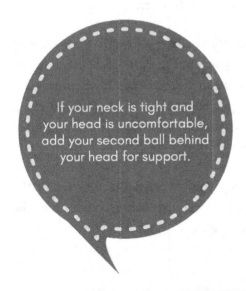

If your neck is tight and your head is uncomfortable, add your second ball behind your head for support.

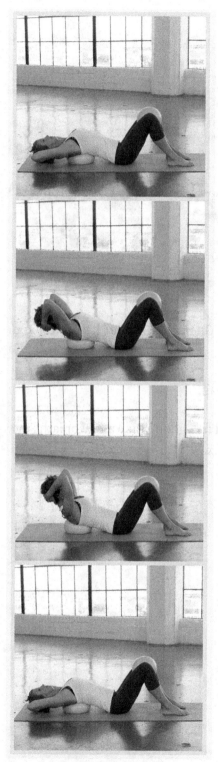

Chest Lift

The directions for all of the variations of the Chest Lift series start the same way as this exercise. I'm not going to repeat the setup portion on the rest of the chest lift exercises because that would bore you!

Place one ball under your upper mid-back, between your shoulder blades.

Place the second ball between your knees, and keep it engaged throughout the exercise.

Interlace your fingers together and place them behind your head. Rest your head in your hands.

As you inhale slowly to the count of four, open your chest, and lie back over the ball. Begin to move your elbows in toward each other.

Slowly exhale through your mouth as you squeeze the ball some more between your knees. Slowly press your upper back into the ball while lifting your chest. Make sure you exhale all of the air out.

Keep your eyes gazing forward at the ball between your knees (not up to the ceiling).

Pause and pull your lower abdominals deeper in and up under your rib cage for four counts.

Relax back over the ball to stretch your chest and belly.

Repeat five to ten times.

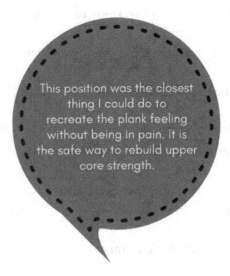

This position was the closest thing I could do to recreate the plank feeling without being in pain. It is the safe way to rebuild upper core strength.

Chest Lift and Lower Core Combination

Start with the Chest Lift setup.

Exhale, curl your tailbone toward your pubic bone, and move into a pelvic tilt. You will feel your lower back connect to the floor.

Enjoy the stretch in your lower back. Relax and breathe.

Exhale and relax your pelvis back into a neutral position in four counts.

Inhale and slowly stretch back over the ball in four counts.

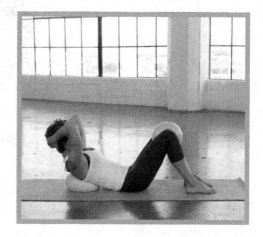

Rest and enjoy the chest and belly stretch.

Repeat five to ten times.

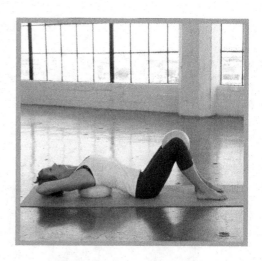

Single-Knee Levitation (Upper Core)

Place the ball under your back, between your shoulder blades.

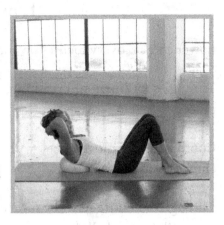

Single knee levitation

Press your upper back into the ball until you feel your upper abdominals engage.

Inhale and curl your tailbone towards your pubic bone to engage your lower abdominals.

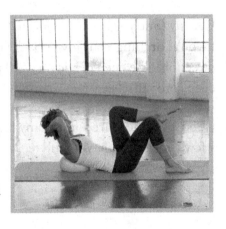

Exhale and slowly lift your right knee. Press your left foot into the floor to connect your core muscles deeper.

Slowly lower your leg in four counts without moving your pelvis.

Do five to ten repetitions on one leg and switch sides.

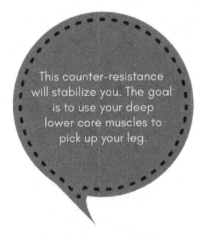

This counter-resistance will stabilize you. The goal is to use your deep lower core muscles to pick up your leg.

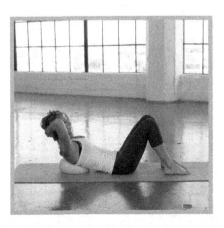

Lower Core

Lower core recovery focuses on your lower body, from the navel down.

Timing, coordination, breathing, and patience are all important to the process.

Coordinate all movements with the breath—and **slow** down. I can't emphasize that enough.

Through this entire series be sure to keep reminding yourself to stay in your pelvic tilt on the ball. It makes a huge difference in the way you feel your lower core muscles.

If at any time you feel disconnected to your core, simply tilt your pelvis more. If you're arching your lower back you are moving your pelvis in the wrong direction. The deep pelvic tilt at all times on this ball will help activate your deep core muscles.

Good luck, these are some of my favorite exercises! If you can practice these a few times a week, you will feel a difference in a very short time.

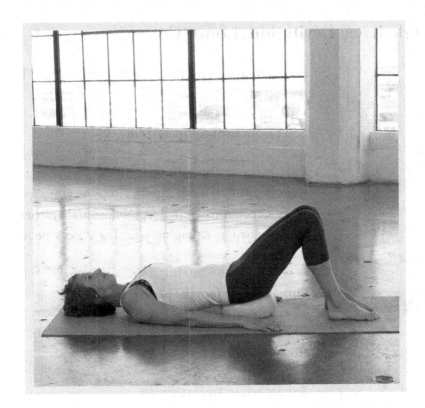

Basic Pelvic Tilt on Ball

Lift hips and place the ball under your pelvis.

Curl your tailbone toward your pubic bone, moving yourself into the pelvic tilt. You will feel your lower abdominals engaged, especially across the lower pelvic region.

Sink your feet into the floor. This allows you to connect deeper to your core muscles.

Do not arch your back or let your abdominals bulge out.

This is the basic movement you will use for the entire lower core series.

It will help you maintain a deeper connection to your lower abdominals.

Single Knee Levitation (Lower Core)

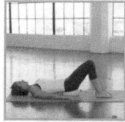
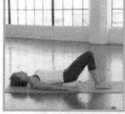

(*Levitation* refers to a slow lift of a "heavy-weighted" leg.)

Start from the basic pelvic tilt.

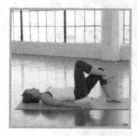

Exhale gently through your mouth and levitate your right leg in four slow counts. Imagine you are lifting your knee from your deep abdominals rather than using your leg. (Imagine your leg is very heavy and hard to lift.)

Sink your left foot deeper into the floor.

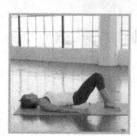

Exhale and lower your leg slowly in a four count. (Keep pelvic tilt.)

Repeat ten to twenty times.

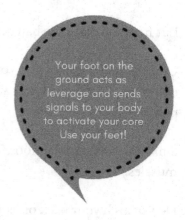

Your foot on the ground acts as leverage and sends signals to your body to activate your core. Use your feet!

Single Knee Levitations with Push to Straight Leg

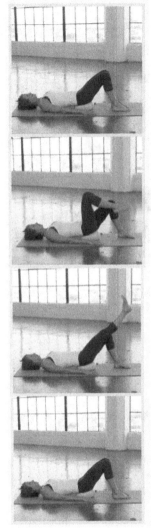

Single Knee Levitations with Push to Straight Leg

Start from basic pelvic tilt.

Exhale gently through your mouth and slowly levitate your knee toward your chest in a slow four count.

Inhale, pause, then exhale as you push your leg out in a straight line.

Inhale and pull the abdominals in even more to bring your knee back to your chest while you exhale and slowly lower your leg back to start position.

Switch to the other leg and repeat.

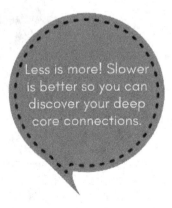

Less is more! Slower is better so you can discover your deep core connections.

Abdominal stretch

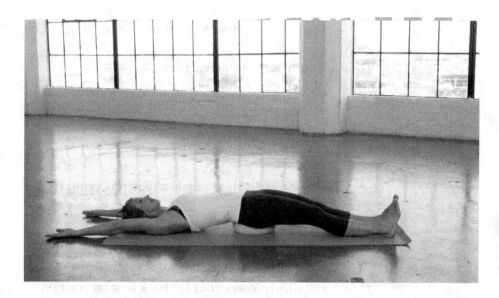

Stretch out over the ball with your arms over your head.

Time to relax and let go.

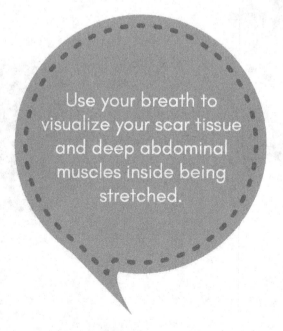

Use your breath to visualize your scar tissue and deep abdominal muscles inside being stretched.

Take Your Core Work
to the Next Level

This section will prepare you for the more advanced strengthening and balancing work coming in the next two phases.

The large stability ball creates an unstable surface, which requires that your core muscles work harder to help you stay balanced.

Note: You will need one 55 inch large stability exercise ball.

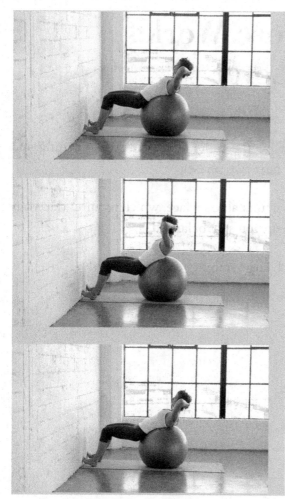

Chest Lifts on Ball

Lie on the ball with your lower back supported and feet firmly planted on the floor.

Interlace your hands behind your head for support. Inhale and prepare.

Exhale gently through your mouth in four slow counts, and slowly lift your trunk up until you feel your core activated.

Inhale and hold for four counts.

Exhale and lower back to start in four slow counts.

The ball is great to support your back so you do not strain.

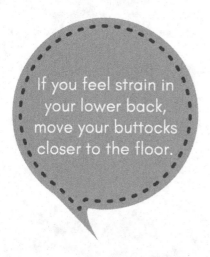

If you feel strain in your lower back, move your buttocks closer to the floor.

Straight Leg Pelvic Bridge Lift

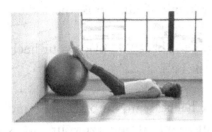

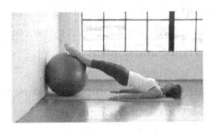

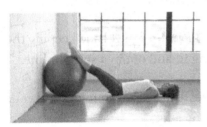

Place your stability ball against the wall.

Lie flat on your back and place your heels on top of the ball.

Press your heels down into the ball and lift your hips off of the ground. Squeeze your butt as you lift. Keep your feet, inner thighs, and hips squeezing together tightly. It helps you maintain balance and control.

Use your arms to help you balance by pressing your palms into the floor.

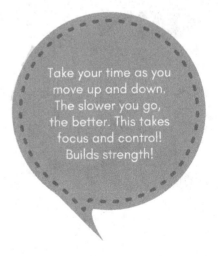

Take your time as you move up and down. The slower you go, the better. This takes focus and control! Builds strength!

Straight Leg Bridge Leg Pulls

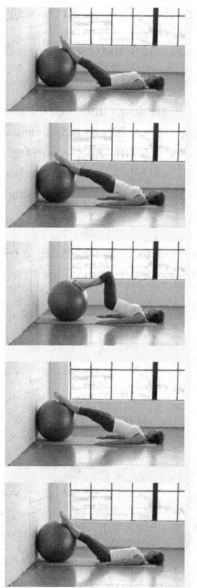

Place your stability ball against the wall.

Lie flat on your back and place your heels on top of the ball.

Press your heels firmly into the ball and begin to lift your hips. Squeeze your butt as you lift. Keep your feet, inner thighs, and hips squeezing together tightly. It helps you maintain balance and control.

Pull the ball toward your hips and pause; then extend your legs straight and lower yourself down to rest.

Keep your focus on control and keeping the ball moving in and out in a straight line.

You will feel the backs of your legs and your butt working a lot!

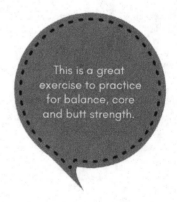

This is a great exercise to practice for balance, core and butt strength.

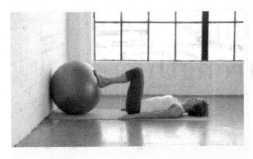

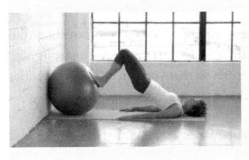

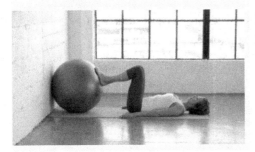

Bridge Lifts

Use a wall for more stability in the beginning. As you gain more strength, you can move away from the wall.

Place your feet on the ball with your knees bent.

The goal is to keep the ball still. Press your feet and heels into the ball to lift your hips up.

Slowly lower your hips back to the ground while keeping the ball still.

This is core, balance, and strength work.

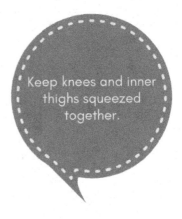

Keep knees and inner thighs squeezed together.

Phase 4: Regaining Balance and Strength

In this phase, you will focus on lower extremity strength, balance and body awareness.

Strength, balance and body awareness are important as you transition into more normal activities of daily living (ADL's). ADL's require strong and balanced muscles in the lower extremities so that you can perform activities such as squatting and balancing (at times on one foot).

Quality is always more important than quantity when practicing these (and any) exercises.

Practice any of the Phase 4 exercises three times per week.

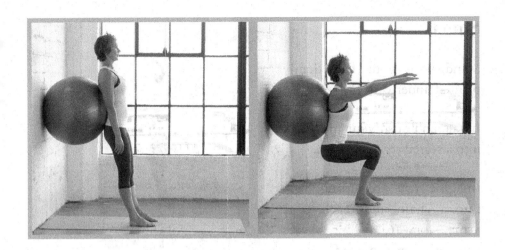

Wall Squats

Place the ball between the wall and your lower back for support. Walk your feet out slightly.

Move your body in a slow four count down toward the floor in a squat position. Imagine you are going to sit down into a chair by pushing back with your hips. Push into the ball with your back to maintain contact. The ball will glide down the wall with you.

If you want to challenge yourself, hold the squat for four counts.

Return to the start position by pushing through your heels.

Start with three to five repetitions, working your way up to ten repetitions.

You can repeat this three times throughout your day.

Squat

Stand with your feet firmly planted under your hips.

Inhale and push your hips back into a seated squat position.

Imagine you are sitting back into a chair, and reach your arms forward. This helps counterbalance yourself.

Exhale and press through your heels and feet to come back to a standing position.

Pressing through your heels activates your "booty" muscles.

Repeat five to ten times and do many times throughout the day.

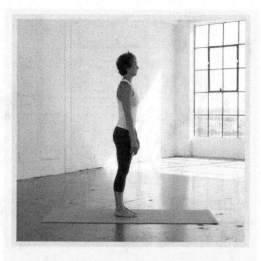

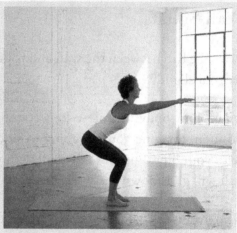

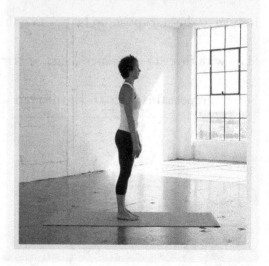

Tree

I recommend standing near a wall when you start practicing Tree pose. A wall never lies and puts you in correct alignment. When you feel more confident, try doing Tree pose without using the wall.

Stand with your feet grounded into the floor and legs together. At first, you can stand next to a wall or hold onto a chair for support.

Slide your right foot up your leg until you find a comfortable spot to hold it on your left, inner leg.

Press your foot and your leg together to create tension. This will help your foot stay in place and not slip down.

If you can balance easily in this position and want to go to the next step, join your palms at the center of your chest.

Then, slowly stretch your arms up toward the ceiling.

The pictures show modifications. If your shoulders are tight, spread your arms wide.

Repeat this mantra in the pose: I am strong, I am balanced and I am determined.

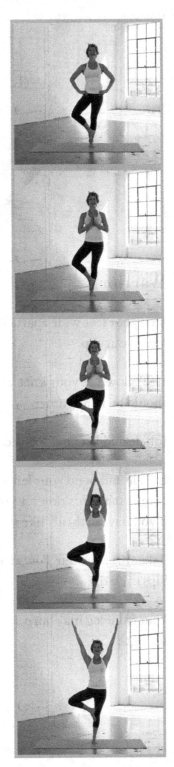

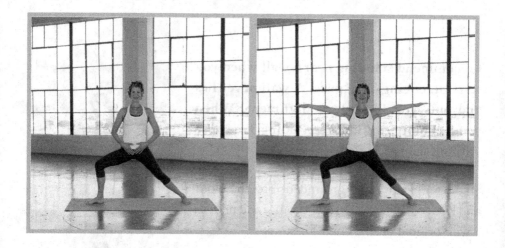

Warrior 2

Step your feet wide apart. Turn your right foot inward and your left foot out from your hip.

Look down at your knee and foot on the front leg. Your foot, hip, and knee should be in alignment.

Inhale and lift your arms out to the side.

Exhale and bend your left knee, sinking and relaxing your hips down into a comfortable position for your hips (the ultimate goal is ninety degrees, but if you have arthritis like me, don't push it).

Take three or four slow, deep breaths in and out, relaxing deeper into your hips each time.

Your front leg may burn a little, but don't worry. That means you're building strength!

Phase 5: Advanced Balance and Strengthening

Phase 5 is a progression of Phase 4, focusing on more complex exercises for strength, balance and body awareness. These are some of my favorite exercises that I *still* do to this day.

I recommend having a chair close by to hold on to for balance. Once you feel confident and strong, you can practice without the chair.

People often think that because they are using a prop, like a chair or wall, that it must mean that the exercise is going to be easy. I disagree. **I live by the motto, less is more.** What this means is that it is important to set your intention with each and every exercise.

In this phase, your intention is building strength to support your bones and joints. I'm sure you've experienced how your quality of life is affected after cancer treatments. You may experience osteoporosis or weakness in your body. By practicing these exercises carefully and with intention, you will regain overall strength and confidence in your body.

Have fun!

I recommend practicing five really good repetitions to start out with. For example, when practicing Single Leg Balance Swings, practice five *slow* ones. This is not about speed, but rather quality movement to build overall strength. Hold the chair for five repetitions on each leg. If you feel you are ready to do more, try doing five more without the chair but have it close by just in case. This exercise will challenge every part of you. I love it!

If you catch yourself saying, *"I can't do this,"* remember how far you have come.

You've got this!

Triangle Pose

Step your legs wide apart.

Turn the back left foot and leg in so that your toes and knees face inward. Turn your right leg out from your hips.

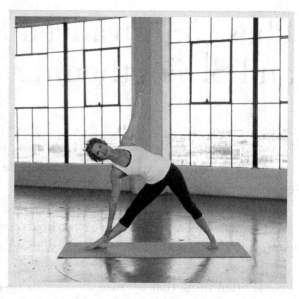

Keep your hands on your hips or reach your arms out to the side. Inhale and pause; then hinge at your hip and push it back to deepen the crease in your right hip.

Exhale and slide your hand down your leg, keeping your spine and back as straight as possible.

It really is one of my favorite standing poses. It targets many muscle groups while it works on strength and flexibility.

It feels so good on the pelvis, legs, and back.

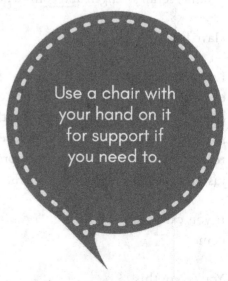

Use a chair with your hand on it for support if you need to.

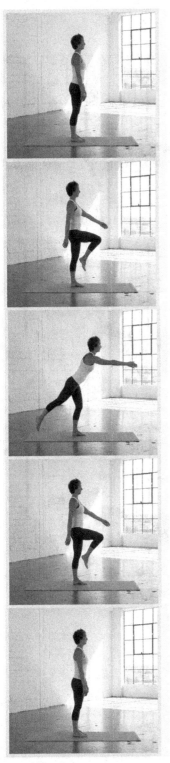

Single Leg Balance Swings

Stand with your feet firmly planted under your hips. Hold a chair if you need support.

Bend and lift your right knee up as you lift your left arm.

Slowly extend your right leg behind you, allowing your left knee to bend slightly. Reach both arms forward for counterbalance.

Pause.

Press through your standing foot to activate your legs, butt, and hips.

Slowly return back to the start position.

Repeat three to five times and change sides.

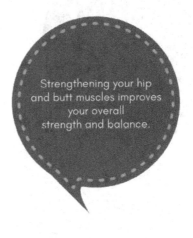

Strengthening your hip and butt muscles improves your overall strength and balance.

Warrior 3

Stand next to your chair and step your feet hip-width apart. Hold the chair for stability in the beginning.

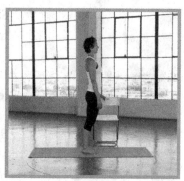

Slowly reach your right arm out in front as you hold the chair with your left hand, and reach your right leg behind you as you hinge forward from your hips in a slow four count.

Slightly bend your standing leg for better balance and strength.

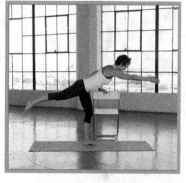

Slowly lower your arm and leg in a slow four count back to the start position.

Turn and repeat on the other side.

More advanced variation: try this exercise without the chair.

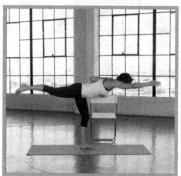

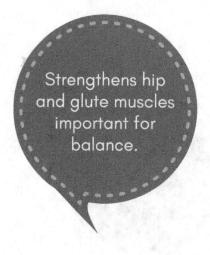

Strengthens hip and glute muscles important for balance.

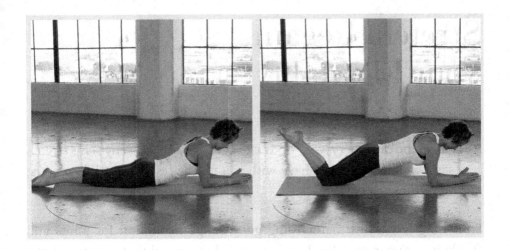

Kneeling Plank

Lie face down with your forearms on the floor and your elbows under your shoulders. Keep your fingers interlaced or palms pressed together.

Bring your feet and knees together and lift your hips off of the floor. This plank is different because the feet, knees, and ankles are squeezing together. This action targets your lower core while taking strain off of your neck and shoulders.

Once in the position, go through these check points:

- Squeeze ankles and feet
- Squeeze knees and inner thighs
- Tighten your hips
- Lift abdominals deeper in and up from your navel area
- Keep rib cage narrowed, no "rib flare"

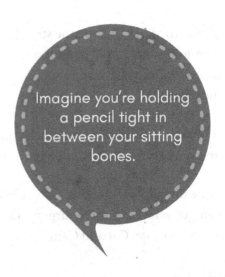

Imagine you're holding a pencil tight in between your sitting bones.

Stretch: Regain Your Flexibility

After any kind of surgery, your body can get tight and feel achy. This stretch series is a wonderful tool to have with you for the rest of your life, not just during your recovery.

Stretching is vital in maintaining good range of motion for joints and flexibility of your muscles. I am sure you have heard that scar tissue can form after any surgery. It's true. These exercises I provide are specifically tailored to those who have had major abdominal and pelvic surgery. You may not expect your hips and back to get tight and sore after surgery, but they do. Your entire body is affected and it's important to love and honor all of you.

Enjoy a stretch today. There is no set number you have to do. I recommend starting with at least three stretches a day. Pick and choose your favorites and you can build yourself up to an entire home practice just from these stretches!

Simple is good. Less is more. Focus on proper technique and form and most importantly, listen to your body.

These are deep, therapeutic stretches that can be held from 30 to 90 seconds. The longer you hold each stretch, the more likely your body will let go of fears, and your scar tissue in and around your abdomen and hips will loosen up.

Remember, your core is so much more than you think. Refer back to the core anatomy section to review what area of muscles you will be focusing on.

For example, in Kneeling Gate it helps to stretch your psoas muscle which can get very tight after surgery. Downward Dog helps with digestion and so much more. Cat and Camel Stretch helps with the mobility of your joints and helps stretch your tight belly muscles. Sitting Wide Legs and Sitting Frog help relax and stretch your pelvic floor.

Each stretch was designed with you and your recovery in mind. I know because I created it at my worst, when my body was in the most pain. I know it works and hope you don't think of this as just another yoga stretch.

These stretches were made with love just for you!

Child's Pose

Begin on your hands and knees. Spread your knees wide apart while keeping your big toes touching. Sit back and rest your buttocks on your heels.

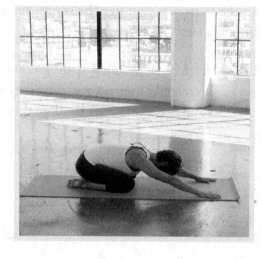

Your ribs and chest should rest comfortably between your legs.

Keep your arms long and extended, palms facing down. Press into the floor with your hands to stretch your skin from your fingers all the way to your toes.

Turn your awareness inward. Begin to let your thoughts slow down. Breathe in relaxation, and exhale tension.

Hold for up to a minute or longer.

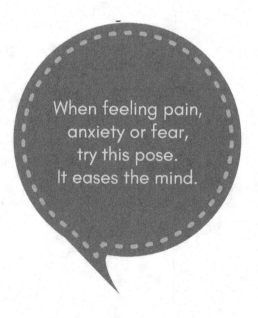

When feeling pain, anxiety or fear, try this pose. It eases the mind.

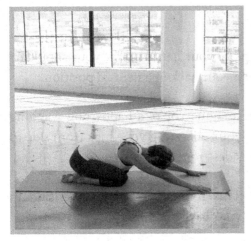

Side Reach

Start in Child's Pose.

Walk your hands to your right side on a diagonal. Go for the biggest stretch of your side waist here by stretching your left arm farther past your right hand.

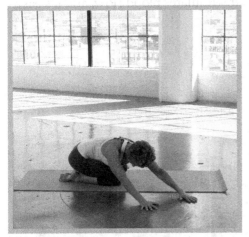

Press your hands into the floor, creating resistance. This helps to increase the stretch.

You should feel your skin stretching all the way from your fingertips to your armpits, through your back and waist.

Breathe into your rib cage and imagine a balloon expanding. This stretches the little muscles in between the ribs and exercises the lungs.

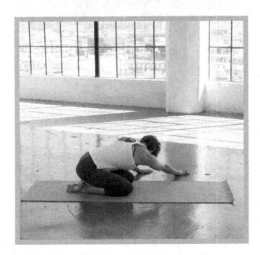

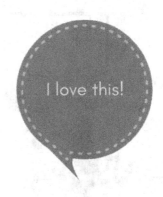

I love this!

Wag the Dog

Come onto your hands and knees; place your hands under your shoulders and your knees under your hips. Keep your back in a neutral position.

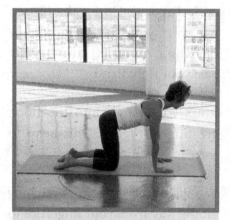

Imagine you're a happy dog wagging your tail—wag your hips from side to side!

This movement releases tension in your back and hips.

It stimulates blood flow, and it's easy!

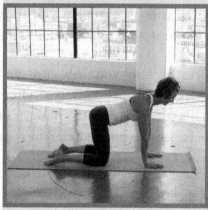

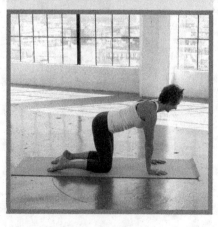

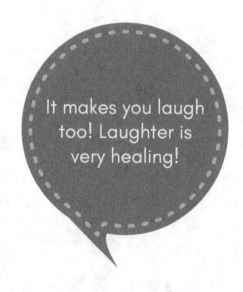

It makes you laugh too! Laughter is very healing!

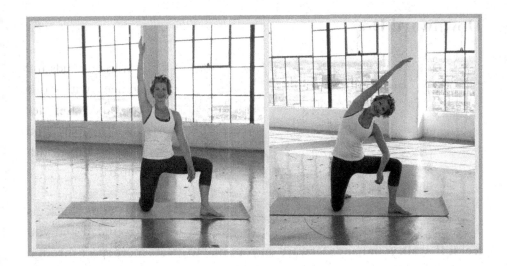

Gate Modified

Kneel down. Move your right leg to the side, forming a right angle of ninety degrees.

Reach your left arm up as you inhale and stretch.

Exhale and slowly reach to the right. Reach just enough to feel a nice stretch on the left side of your waist, lower back, and rib cage.

Place your right forearm on your knee to help support your body.

You can use that arm to create resistance or tension to give you a deeper stretch.

I do this pose three times a day. It's one of my favorite go-to stretches.

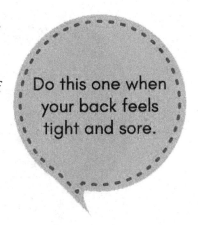

Do this one when your back feels tight and sore.

Downward Dog

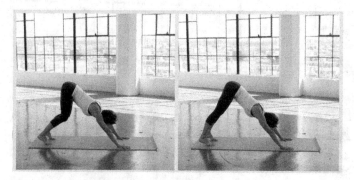

Start on hands and knees with your hands shoulder width apart and knees hip width apart.

If your back is rounded and you feel stiff, walk your hands forward on your mat to create more space through your spine.

Lift your knees off the floor and keep them bent. Push your hands into the floor and stretch your hips back.

Move your sitting bones up to the ceiling. (This really increases the stretch in your legs.)

Straighten your legs if you can for a full body stretch.

The goal isn't to get your heels to the floor. Just create good body alignment and stretch.

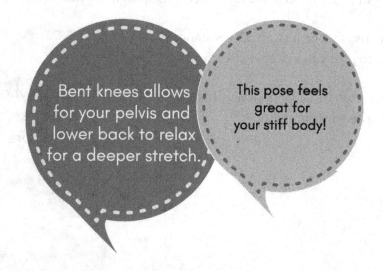

Bent knees allows for your pelvis and lower back to relax for a deeper stretch.

This pose feels great for your stiff body!

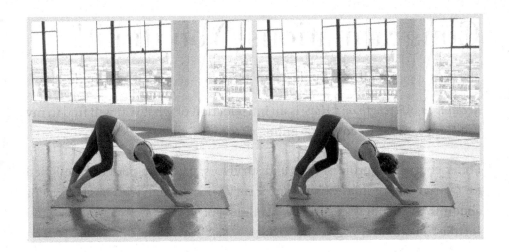

Walk the Dog

Start in Downward Dog. This time you want to focus on getting one heel down to the floor at a time. This creates a deeper stretch in your calf muscles!

Bend your right knee and stretch your left leg straight. Relax your heel down into the floor for a deep stretch.

Breathe and relax here for 30-60 seconds.

Then switch legs.

If your arms get tired, rest in between.

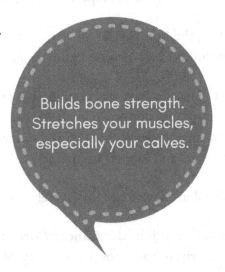

Builds bone strength. Stretches your muscles, especially your calves.

Congratulations! You did it!

Reclaim Your Strength and Hope is an introduction of what you will find in my full **Cancer Core Recovery®** online program.

I offer courses for professionals and survivors. They are perfectly designed for ovarian/abdominal/pelvic cancer survivors, anyone who has had major abdominal and pelvic surgery, wellness professionals, caretakers, and certified Pilates and yoga instructors.

I have so much more goodness for you—over 100 exercises with detailed instructional videos and printable lessons in PDF format. Plus, bonus content to inspire you to work out with me every day.

After you enroll in my full online program, you will have:

- Improved Pelvic Wellness
- Stronger Abdominal Muscles
- Increased Flexibility & Mobility
- Relief From Back Pain & Better Posture and Balance
- Feelings of Peacefulness, Wellbeing, Self-Compassion and Self-Love
- A Sense of Hope and Excitement for the Future

And, the best part of all of this? **The Cancer Core Recovery® Program** includes a 24/7, private online community!

My favorite part of creating this program has been building an online community of women in all stages of cancer recovery! I felt so alone during my own recovery that I vowed to create a space where other women could connect and support each other.

You don't have to do this alone!

When you join the **Cancer Core Recovery® Program**, I'll add you to my private Facebook community of women in cancer recovery, just like you. You'll begin to feel more supported and understood by other women taking this amazing journey. You'll be able to share your struggles and your accomplishments without the fear of being judged or shamed.

And, of course, I will be in the group with you, cheering you on every step of the way! I will share motivational and inspiring ideas, new exercises, nutritional guidance and delicious, healthy recipes every week!

Visit my website at www.emileegarfield.com and be a part of my thriving community of women in cancer recovery!

Love and hugs,
Emilee

About Emilee Garfield

Emilee considers herself a cancer *thriver*–she has recovered from cancer twice and it is her mission to help other cancer survivors live with hope and joy.

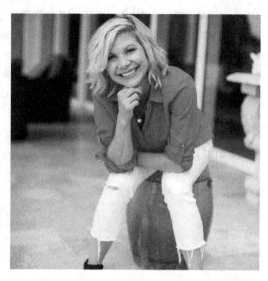

She was first diagnosed at age four with a rare cancer called Rhabdomyosarcoma. After two years of grueling radiation and chemotherapy, she survived. Years later, while in college, Emilee had a partial hysterectomy because she tested positive for pre-cervical cancer.

In 2015, she was diagnosed with Stage 3C ovarian cancer and her battle was the inspiration for her first book, *Reclaim Your Strength and Hope: Exercises for Cancer Core Recovery®*.

This is how her book *Reclaim Your Strength and Hope: Exercises for Cancer Core Recovery* was developed. In order to write the book, she researched and taught herself how to rebuild her strength and flexibility.

Emilee created a library of over 200 gentle movement exercises and stretches to help cancer survivors feel better in their bodies during a time when everything seems like it's falling apart. More than just physical exercises, the book is filled with love and support. Emilee talks to the survivor as if she's right there by their side.

At the time of her recovery from ovarian cancer, Emilee was a single mom with three children and had no choice but to return to work as a Yoga/Pilates instructor as soon as possible, with her new ostomy. There were limited exercise resources available to help her safely rebuild her core muscles, but she knew movement was medicine and that she would heal faster by gently moving her body.

In 2016, Emilee filled that void when she founded The Cancer Core Recovery® Project, a non-profit, 501 (c)(3) foundation that provides educational exercise programs, workout videos and instructional training manuals to help survivors of ovarian cancer enjoy a better quality of life.

Emilee has been teaching yoga and pilates for the past 21 years at her studio, The Loft, in Santa Barbara, California. She is a professional life coach, a certified New Life Story® coach and her passion is helping women reclaim their strength and hope using movement as medicine.

You can learn more about how to work with Emilee on her website: www.emileegarfield.com

Printed in the United States
By Bookmasters